Praise for *Body Thrive*

"In *Body Thrive*, Cate Stillman expertly distills the time-tested and often complex wisdom of Ayurveda to provide succinct tools and practical daily habits to help modern humans experience extraordinary health. This is the next frontier of Ayurveda."

> MARK HYMAN, MD
> medical director at Cleveland Clinic's Center for Functional
> Medicine and 11-time #1 *New York Times* bestselling author.

"Ayurveda is not only ancient Indian medicine—it is a universal body of knowledge that Cate Stillman delivers seamlessly into your living room, where it belongs. *Body Thrive* offers Ayurvedic practices that are doable and logical for modern readers!"

> JOHN DOUILLARD, DC, CAP
> bestselling author, founder of LifeSpa.com

"In *Body Thrive*, Cate Stillman delivers the timeless, ancient wisdom of Ayurveda in a practical 10-step program. Within the thalamus part of the brain, there is a special gene which maintains the circadian rhythms of our biological clock. Stillman's teachings touch this subtle, invisible clock, bringing harmony, happiness, and long life. This book will change your body, mind, and consciousness so your life can become more whole."

> VASANT LAD, BAM&S, MASC
> founder of The Ayurvedic Institute, author of *The*
> *Complete Book of Ayurvedic Home Remedies*

"*Body Thrive* distills a road map for optimal health for the mystery we live in . . . our body. I recommend using Cate's 10 habit principles to get into alignment and to discover your unique purpose in being alive in these interesting, changing times."

> ANA T. FORREST
> creatrix of Forrest Yoga and author of *Fierce Medicine*

"The beauty of the ancient tradition of Ayurveda is that it brings to the forefront the necessity of ritual for the body, mind, and soul. *Body Thrive* is a coming home, a way to truly be present with who we are on the spiritual level, by engaging in body-based self-care practices. This book is the perfect manual for honoring your body as a temple so that your life is manageable, fulfilling, and joyful!"

DEANNA MINICH, PHD
author of *Chakra Foods for Optimum Health* and *The Rainbow Diet*

"As complexity increases all around us, it is easy to forget that the most effective tools we have to make positive changes in ourselves are often the simplest. Change your habits and you change your existence. In *Body Thrive*, Cate Stillman—who has revised basic teachings from Ayurveda to fit the modern world—offers practical tools for realigning our lives with the rhythms of Life that our bodies crave to follow. Make an honest effort to introduce these 10 habits into your existence and you are certain to benefit."

ROBERT SVOBODA
BAMS (Ayurvedacharya), author of *Prakriti: Your Ayurvedic Constitution*

"Cate Stillman is a healer and a dedicated advocate for self-healing through yoga and Ayurveda. In these pages, you will learn to nurture and nourish yourself by attuning your habits to focus on positive choices that garner health and happiness."

MAYA TIWARI
Ayurveda pioneer, author, and humanitarian

"How many of us struggle with the wide chasm between what we *know* is ideal health and what we *do* to achieve it? In *Body Thrive*, Cate Stillman has distilled her decades of education and experience leading thousands through exemplary programs that build this bridge. She takes you through a powerful program with 10 simple but potent habits so that you can truly thrive."

ERIC GRASSER, MD, CAY

"*Body Thrive* engages readers with life-changing advice and a no-nonsense approach to lasting health. I love how Cate ushers her readers into taking action so that they too can be masters of Ayurveda."

TALYA LUTZKER
author of *The Ayurvedic Vegan Kitchen*

"In *Body Thrive*, Cate Stillman has provided a manifesto to thrive—not just survive—in our lives. Packed with numerous actionable pearls of wisdom for optimizing sleep, nutrition, movement, and connection with self and others, you can feel Cate's approach to a body-empowered and zestful life come through the pages!"

MARK MENOLASCINO, MD
author of *Heart Solution for Women*

"*Body Thrive* is an upbeat and inspiring take on Ayurvedic wisdom. Cate's supportive and engaging style welcomes readers into the fold and sets us up for success from the very beginning. Creating new habits is indeed an evolutionary science, and Body Thrive is on the cusp of this movement."

KATE O'DONNELL
modern yoga wisdom teacher and author of *The Everyday Ayurveda Cookbook* and *Everyday Ayurveda Cooking for a Calm, Clear Mind*

"Cate is a genius at sharing the potent self-care practices of Ayurveda in an accessible, methodical, and joyful way. *Body Thrive* is an invaluable guide for anyone interested in self-healing and transformation."

SCOTT BLOSSOM
founder of Shunyata Yoga

body
thrive

body thrive

uplevel your body &
your life with 10 habits
from ayurveda & yoga

CATE STILLMAN

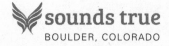

sounds true
BOULDER, COLORADO

Sounds True, Inc.
Boulder, CO 80306

Published 2019
Previously published as *Body Thrive: Uplevel Your Body and Your Life
with 10 Habits from Ayurveda and Yoga*, 2015.

Cover design by Rachael Murray
Book design by Beth Skelley

Printed in Canada

Cataloging-in-Publication data for this book is available from the Library of Congress.
ISBN: 978-1-68364-262-6 (pbk.)
ISBN: 978-1-68364-338-8 (ebook)

10 9 8 7 6 5 4 3 2 1

To the Planet

May we humans awaken to our potentials of dynamic collaboration with each other and with Earth.

To My Clients

To the certified coaches in the worldwide association of Yoga Health Coaching and to the Body Thrive Coaches for your studentship (*adhikara*) and your dharma. May this book help you help others as you set the global standard for Yoga Health Coaching.

To My Teachers' Teachers

I'm a synthesizer. My tremendous teachers imparted deep wisdom, and I attempt to make this wisdom even more user friendly. In this book, you may recognize the voices of my teachers. They are, in order of appearance in my life: Tim and Missy Goss, Don Cannon, professor Michael Molitor, John Friend, Dr. Vasant Lad, Sally Kempton, Craig Hamilton, Katrina Blair, and Dr. Claudia Welch. In gratitude to all those who dedicate their life to seeking, living, and sharing deep wisdom for the good of all.

Contents

You Only Get One Body

You only get one body. Which habits are you going to mold it with?

There is a rhythm to your body thriving. When you know and live into this rhythm, you engage in your best life ever. The rhythm creates an order. When you engage the order, you thrive; when you disregard it, you suffer.

This suffering may be slow and superficial, or deep and painful. The aim of this book is to up your thrive through engaging the rhythm of life, the natural order.

A vibrant physique, an abundance of energy, and higher consciousness are worthy aims for the arrow of your attention.

Ayurveda, an age-old science of rejuvenation, gives you a manual for body wisdom and daily thrive as you chronologically age. If you up your game in wellness and body smarts by learning from your yesterdays, you experience body thrive. Learning from past behavior is the basis of health and healing. Informed, intentional habits rejuvenate you.

Part 1

Orientation

How Are You Designing Your Body?

Your reality in body, mind, and spirit is a reflection of your habits. Your choices heal or undermine you, and your habits direct the lens through which you view your life. These small, seemingly inconsequential habits breed your life experience. Will you merely survive? Or earnestly thrive? Better habits open and strengthen your body even as you age; they open your mind to attract ideas that align with what you want to do and who you want to become next. Better habits also awaken your spirit and foster better relationships.

If your current habits are aggravating your body but you keep up your current state of affairs, you'll exacerbate those aggravations, and things will get worse. When you don't act on what you've learned, you turn your direction toward suffering, which leads to aging. You'll be grumpy, anxious, tired, stiff, or fat instead of fluid, graceful, fun, and sparky.

You craft your inner universe: how it's organized, how it runs, the vibe, and the way you age. What is the organization of your organism? How is your reverberation? Are you fluid, connected, contented? Or are you chaotic, stressed, overscheduled, bloated, or depleted? Are your habits intentional and effortful, or careless and regressive?

Your Habits Should Get Smarter as You Age

As a self-reflective human, you're designed to get smarter. By your very design, you can upgrade how you experience your life by refining, reforming, and then automating your habits. Right now, you are choosing the habits that will generate future ease or future stress.

When you slip into substandard habits, you start to live out of sync. Your emotions will generate a negative reverberation, which will, in turn, influence your thoughts and your biochemistry. You will experience more stress than ease in your emotions, in your thoughts, in your relationships, and in your body.

In this book, I crack the code of ten essential daily habits from the deep and ancient holistic science of Ayurveda, the perennial body-wisdom tradition that arose in tandem with yoga, the fully embodied path of living awake and at ease. Here lies a simple curriculum that every person should learn as a child, master as an adult, and refine as an elder for their body and life to thrive. *Body Thrive* is about upleveling your habits into the habits of ease, of wellness, of thrive.

The Wisdom of Yogis Is Based on Habits

The yogis of yore deeply explored human consciousness. Through their four-plus millennia of guru-to-disciple personal experimentation, the *yogis* (yoga masters) and *vaidyas* (Ayurvedic doctors and masters) discovered that consciousness in both mind and spirit is wired through physiology.

Matter equals energy. As you open and strengthen the body's subtle energy technology, you open the mind to higher thought. You open your emotions to bliss and interconnectivity. Your physical body can support the capacity of your spirit to expand, and vice versa. As you pulsate, building integrity on both the subtle and gross levels, your capacity for thrive amplifies.

The body is wired for ecstasy, what the yogis call *bliss*. Your biochemistry is your pharmacology. The ten Body Thrive practices from yoga and Ayurveda teach you how to turn on and subtly optimize your biochemistry and activate your pharmacology. The practices become habits. When you age with the practices of yoga and Ayurveda, you elevate your capacity for and refinement of bliss on all levels of your being: physical, mental, emotional, relational, spiritual. The ecstasy is actually internal—better named "enstacy."

Inversely, most modern humans miss the boat and age themselves with physical, mental, emotional, or relational degeneration, much of which is preventable. We know from Sir Isaac Newton that an object in motion stays in motion with the same speed and in the same direction unless acted upon by another force. Humans are the evolution of the laws of physics and nature. We can consciously choose to align with these laws, which lead to an experience of ease, flow, and the awakened regenerative nature of our bodily intelligence. When we consciously or unconsciously choose not to align with the laws of nature, we suffer the consequence of degeneration.

Ayurveda is based on living in sync. In Ayurveda, the synchronized daily bodily rhythms are called *dinacharya*, which means "following the rhythm of the day." Isn't that lovely? You get to follow; no need to lead. No need for absolutes or rules or internal wars. Just pay attention and follow the lead. Nature isn't just on your side; she's got your back. Dinacharya becomes your daily schedule based on nature's rhythms. When you synchronize your bodily rhythms to nature's clock, your physiology harmonizes. You experience balance, ease, and flow. When you live against nature's body clock, you experience stress, rapid aging, and dis-ease.

Body Thrive ushers its initiates toward subtle alignment with bio-rhythms at the speed of light, or one habit per week. As you drop into the ten core habits that align your day-to-day routine with natural rhythms, you thrive. You become a vibrant, dynamic human being on a growth path, which is a boon to yourself, your family, society, and the planet. You attune to the magnetic pull of the universal energies to align your personal body rhythms—like sleeping, pooping, eating, moving, playing, chillaxing. When you integrate the 10 Habits of Body Thrive, you align with the force of nature. You make the switch from degenerative to regenerative habits. That's a big deal. You win big in the short run. You win bigger in the long run. You design your direction in life. You downshift aging. You evolve physically, relationally, and emotionally. This may sound like a tall order, but rest assured, the teachings in this book are simple, time-tested, empowered practical wisdom.

What Body Thrivers Report

The Body Thrive method came from my search as an innovative Ayurvedic practitioner and yoga teacher for a more effective path to guide my clients toward their desired health breakthroughs and wellness goals. This book grew out of my online Body Thrive coaching program, where my Body Thrive Coaches and Yoga Health Coaches guide members through ten habits in ten weeks. As you'll see, Body Thrive is innovative, practical, and focused on results, which are breathtaking. Actually, the results are breath*giving*. Participants step into the driver's seat of their lives to achieve their ideal body weight, natural rhythm, joy, and enthusiasm. Here are a few of the reports:

> "At the end of the ten weeks, I was surprised to get on the scale and find I was thirty pounds lighter. All I did was master the first habit—an earlier, lighter dinner."

> "I'm now able to get a good night's rest consistently. I can feel my immune system rebuilding. This is a big deal for me as I've struggled with chronic fatigue syndrome for twenty years."

> "I'm finally in control of how I feel. Instead of waking up groggy and grumpy, I wake up clear, alert, and ready for action."

> "I wish I had learned this as a child. I wish my parents had lived these basic habits. My children did this course with me. Our household is running smoother than ever and we're all happier. Amazing."

Body Thrivers evolve into a state of integrity with themselves. Common feedback after ten weeks includes:

- I have more energy.
- I sleep better.
- I eat a healthier diet.
- I've developed better self-care habits.

- I've learned the daily habits for longevity and healthy aging.
- I've started a home yoga practice.
- I've taken my yoga practice deeper.
- I've started meditating.
- I have a stronger, more consistent meditation practice.

I designed the 10 Habits of Body Thrive to help you unwind imbalances in your body-mind that you've generated by living out of sync with your human biorhythms. Experiment with these habits to see how many of the listed results you experience—and how quickly!

After participating in the program, Body Thrivers commonly reflect on imbalances they suffered unnecessarily for years. Through embedding the habits based on humanity's ancient deep rhythms, Body Thrivers are crystal clear about which old habits fed their symptoms, thereby accelerating aging and disease. Able to pilot their own ships, they now steer in the direction they want to go.

There are currently more than a hundred Yoga Health Coaches using the Body Thrive method around the world. A poll of 150 clients showed the following after ten weeks:

- 89 percent developed better self-care habits
- 79 percent feel better in their bodies
- 59 percent are eating a healthier diet
- 51 percent are sleeping better and feel well-rested

I'm not going to ask you to change anything overnight, or even to stop the habits you know aren't helping you. I'm going to nudge you in the right direction for aging in your own skin. Within ten weeks, you will get a solid start. Then I recommend doing Body Thrive again and again and again, one chapter per week. Soon you'll be living the habits and compounding positive benefits to your present and future health.

My History with the Body Thrive Habits

I wrote this book, in part, because I wish I had been raised on Body Thrive. I'm blessed to come from a healthy, active, fun, and athletic family; however, I was not a body-thriving kind of kid. My earliest memories include constipation and migraines. At five years old, I had headaches so bad that they would last three to four consecutive days of every month. Crying made the pain worse, so I learned early on not to cry. The doctors I went to for headaches never asked about the constipation.

It was the late 1970s in America. My childhood community didn't know about holistic wellness. Modern medicine couldn't help me. By my teen years, allergies piled onto the mix of constipation and headaches. The doctors prescribed more pills. My dad nicknamed me "The Pill Popper," and I hoped my chronic body issues would just go away. They didn't. Had my family not been athletic, and had my mom not prepared our meals, my health would have been far worse.

In high school and college, I took the care of my body into my own hands. I experimented with diet. After college, I researched human consciousness, human development, and healing systems. I kept running into Ayurveda. I went to Ayurveda school, and while there, I started to detox my body. The constipation, migraines, and allergies dematerialized. I started to experience empowerment over how I could feel. The old patterns of imbalance became self-evident. This map of habits-symptoms-alleviation was a pivotal breakthrough.

Fast-forward through twenty years of schooling and working as an Ayurvedic practitioner and yoga teacher. In the process of my work, I realized that most of my clients needed to detoxify their habits. I witnessed that my clients who invested in Body Thrive education, guidance, and coaching—the "nuts and bolts" of Ayurveda—had a more rapid and lasting wellness evolution than those who preferred one-to-one treatment with specialized diets, herbal drugs, and body therapies. I've found that my clients and students are more likely to hit their body, mind, and spirit wellness goals when they are part of a community of others working on similar goals.

Finding What Works and Taking Action

This book is the result of a teaching curriculum co-created out of the dynamic micro–think tank and practice lab that includes my clients, students, and colleagues—my tribe. These peeps gave steady feedback about what they wanted next and what wasn't working in their busy lives. My tribe helped me refine the process you'll find in this book. I'm grateful to the innovative community at my wellness hub, Yogahealer.com, which demanded and digested this body of work, and to the certified Yoga Health Coaches for spreading it through their hoods around the planet. Based on this practice lab, the three key components we've found that accelerate wellness evolution are:

1. **Ayurveda**   The habits of Ayurveda, based on biorhythms, are nonnegotiable for thrive. As we align with our biorhythms, we detox our habits. In doing so, our bodies, minds, emotions, and even our kitchens, homes, relationships, and lives uplevel into thrive. We experience the best time of our lives by living in cooperation with our bodies and our ecosystem.

2. **Behavioral science**   Knowing what you *should* do and actually doing it are different sides of the coin. Behavioral science—or what I like to call the science of habit evolution—is what makes Body Thrive effective. Setbacks disappear with a strong, clear intention; smaller steps; tracking; rewards; and conscious community. With these, you will become the person who has the habits of thrive.

3. **Dynamic groups and relationship evolution**   People in groups adopt Body Thrive Habits faster because they're with others who are focusing on similar goals. This book outlines how to create dynamic supportive relationships on the path to daily habit evolution.

These habits are as old as your ancestral lineage. My goal is to help you understand *why* you need them and *how* to embed them into your modern life. Your habits are moldable and become who you are and how you age. Let's see how good you can feel as you design your life intentionally. To do so, I've developed seven keys to help you get the most out of this book:

1. Work one habit a week. Some habits you may already have dialed into. Use those weeks to keep implementing the habits that are edgy for you right now. Don't work at mastery; keep moving forward.

2. Take small actions. Go baby step by baby step, microchoice by microchoice, and keep moving forward. Repetition is the route. Go to bodythrive.com/free to download the free *Body Thrive Workbook*, and print out the worksheets. Use them. They will help you take action.

3. Find a friend. If you're serious about wanting your body to thrive, look for a friend or posse to partner with on the expedition into Body Thrive. A *posse* is a group gathered for a common purpose. Your posse may be one to three friends who want a shift from their tired, overwhelmed, overweight, or inflamed reality. Ask everyone to get their own copy of this book, then commit to each other, the ten-week timeline, and the process. Follow the guidelines in "Create a Book Club for *Body Thrive*" on page 227. Or come to bodythrive.com and join our next live coaching group. Of course, you can go through the book alone. However, being in a group will help you gain deeper traction no matter where you're starting.

4. Follow your desire in how you shift your habits. Your desire is smart. Let it lead the way.

5. Work on what's working. When you get stuck or a habit is particularly unappealing, don't sweat it. Plan on going through the book again after your first ten weeks are done and catching it next time. Body Thrive members repeat the course again and again and again because their lives keep getting better.

6. Do Body Thrive four times a year. Keep cycling through the ten habits every ten weeks. These biorhythmic habits align you with your natural state of perpetual growth and evolution. This book is packed with information so that you can go deeper and learn more with each turn of the wheel.

7. If you want to get started right away, you can skip ahead to Habit 1: Eat an Earlier, Lighter Dinner. When you're ready for the theory and science pieces, come back to this orientation section in part I. The theory and science help, but each chapter stands on its own as well.

As you shape yourself through your habits into a healthy, whole, and interconnected human being on a growth path, you'll notice that people—your family, your community—and even your ecosystem follow your lead. This is an invitation to step into Body Thrive for your personal health *and* for the bigger whole that you are a part of.

Go ahead, spin through the wheel of time with cyclical daily habits that enable you to thrive. Embed better habits, and your day-to-day life will open up. You will live your life more awake, more in light than in darkness.

How to Have a Body
According to Ayurveda

Body *Thrive* is not about magical elixirs or expensive super-foods. The force that will sculpt and shape your body and how you age is daily *habit*.

Maybe habit doesn't sound enticing. Maybe dread quietly appears when you hear the word *habit*. I've seen enough people get their mojo back after years of struggling, and I know one thing for sure: the habits you choose over time create your day-to-day thrive. Your habits also determine your future day-in and day-out experience, for better or worse. As William Durant writes in his interpretation of Aristotle's teachings, "We are what we repeatedly do. Excellence, then, is not an act, but a habit."[1]

Will your current habits beget the future body you desire to live in? Are you evolving and refining your habits as you get older and wiser? Will your habits create cultural and even epigenetic positive momentum for future generations to step into thriving health and easy self-care? When your habits reflect your evolving wisdom, you experience habit evolution. The Sanskrit word that gives insight into this process is *vinayam*.

If you make your own sauerkraut, you understand culture. Like an extended marinade, culturing is a powerful transformation that happens given the right circumstances and time. In this ultimate slow-food method, juice and flavor evolve with age. Vinayam is considered the cultured mannerism that results from your discipline and training. Slow-cooked (or cultured) habits, based on deepening your body wisdom, are your aim. When you slowly culture your repetitive actions as you age, with humble discipline, you are entering the realm of vinayam.

Similar to making sauerkraut, you hit stages of ripening. When the juice and flavor is how you want it, you move your crock to the fridge to stabilize and preserve the flavor. The kraut will continue to culture, more slowly and deeply. So it is with habit evolution. When your learning continuously influences what you choose to do next, you are living vinayam. You don't shut down as you grow older. You wake up.

Cultured Habits + Repetition = Optimal Lifestyle Design

You hold the power to design your body and your life. To uplevel your body, your dharma (or purpose), and your life, you not only need specific habits, you need to *repeat them over time.*

Cup of coffee Monday, cup of coffee Tuesday, cup of coffee Wednesday, and so on, 365 days times fifty years. What is the effect on your kidneys? Your skin? Your nerves and stamina? Instead, replace the coffee with a fresh green juice—or at least have your green juice with your coffee. What is the effect on your kidneys? On your sleep? Your emotions? On how you show up in relationships? If you never transition your habits to those that support thrive, you will never know their cost.

Another Sanskrit word that can help you here is *abhyasa,* an intentional, repetitive practice done for spiritual evolution or long-term gain. Dropping a regressive habit and integrating a progressive habit always involves abhyasa. As your habits evolve consistently through cultured improvement, you build momentum in designing the life and body you want.

How do you evolve? You experiment. Get curious. Curiosity is the necessary stance for habit evolution. Step into your personal biochemistry lab to optimize your body, your mind, and your emotional, relational, and spiritual experience. Humans are designed to learn from experience. When you do, you make better choices. When you don't, you devolve and suffer.

If you want to enjoy your body more, listen to your body. Slow down to feel your emotions, acknowledge signals of fatigue, recognize which foods work for your body, and listen for signals to move or rest. Reflection and better decisions—that is where you start. Become the sovereign of cause and effect.

In yoga, we call the cause-effect cycle *karma*. Karma is the residue—the effect—created from an action. Forces come in pairs. Physicist Isaac Newton postulated that every action has an equal and opposite reaction in both size and direction. Your personal biochem lab is not exempt from this law. If the reaction is desired, repeat the action or even improve upon it. If the reaction is not desired, avoid re-creating the experiment or experience. The key to experimentation is to digest what you've learned and then improve the next experiment. This is a recurring theme to design a better future for yourself.

Informed, Intended Actions and Listening

Every habit carries an energy or intention. As the Bible's Galatians 6:7 says, "As ye sow, so also shall ye reap." You don't just want habits, you want *informed, intended actions* that cultivate deep, consistent momentum toward your desired experiences. Reflection and conscious decision-making are crucial tools for developing informed habits.

The other critical tool is listening for feedback. To thrive, you must listen. Slow down to feel, acknowledge the signals of fatigue, recognize the signals informing you which foods work best for your body, and heed the signals to move or rest. Trust builds as you listen. You'll make decisions that are connected to what you know and how you feel.

When you don't make space to listen or time to feel, and when you disregard your needs, you lose integrity with yourself. If you ignore your body, you lose its trust. When you ignore negative feed-back from your body, emotions, and thought patterns, you lose the opportunity to pivot. If you don't make a decision to change course, you erode your integrity with your body. You inhibit your capacity to listen to your deeper desires. You get stuck or unwell.

The 10 Daily Habits of Body Thrive are simple hygiene practices that give you a structure to listen to your body and guide you toward your sacred, awake, vibrant life. Anyone can become a master. You will become increasingly sensitive to the steady stream of physical, mental, and emotional signals your body emits to help you optimize your energy, your sleep, and your life.

When your habits are out of alignment with time, your body shifts from ease to dis-ease. *Dis-* means "having a negative or reversing force." *Ease* means "free from difficulty, effort, or trouble." Dis-ease, therefore, is reversing the flow of ease. Dis-ease is disease. Behaviors that reverse the flow of ease beget disease. Ayurveda names three causes of disease:

- *prajnaparadha*: making negligent choices
- *asatmendriyartha samyoga*: disrespecting your senses
- *parinama*: the process or movement of time

The causes of disease describe the negative feedback loop of dishonoring what you've learned, which leads to craving what hurts you, which further leads to getting out of sync with the universe. Oy vey. When you understand the three causes, you get an owner's manual to thriving through your wisdom years.

CAUSE OF DISEASE #1   Making Careless Choices

Negligence is not applying intelligence, not applying common sense, or flat-out disregarding what you already know. *Prajnaparadha* refers to not learning from your experience. Poor choices piled up on each other lead to unclear thinking and unintelligent cravings, which lead to even poorer choices. Take a moment to pause and reflect on this. Most of humanity can relate to prajnaparadha on some level. Can you?

Your intelligence detector, named *prajna*, is inborn. And violable. When you violate yourself by disregarding what you've learned from experience, you suffer. Thus, the first cause of disease is offending yourself, trespassing against yourself, hurting yourself by not correcting behavior today based on what you know from your yesterdays. We all fall into this trap.

CAUSE OF DISEASE #2 Disrespecting Your Senses

Let's take apart the lengthy Sanskrit word for "disrespecting your senses": asatmendriyartha samyoga. *Astmaya* means "inappropriate," *indriya* means "sense organs," *artha* means "the objects of the senses," and *samyoga* means "to combine" or "to link."

Your senses are delicate instruments able to discriminate between delight and damage. Pay very close attention to what you taste, see, hear, feel, and smell. What delights and nurtures your senses? Tune in to your senses to find out. Your senses will tell you when they've had enough. Your job is to pay attention and respond appropriately.

When you make inappropriate choices repetitively, you confuse or damage your senses. Confusion blocks the flow of consciousness. Damage destroys consciousness. Making decisions from a place of unconsciousness will destroy you over time. That is the teaching behind asatmendriyartha samyoga.

Be attentive to your body: detect when music is too aggressive, food is too processed, or your eyes are too tired to read the screen. If you disrespect your senses, you cause disease in your body, your mind, your relationships, and your spiritual life. Respect the wisdom and sensitivity of your senses.

CAUSE OF DISEASE #3 Accelerating Aging by Living Out of Rhythm with the Cosmic Clock

The third cause of disease—the way to sink your ship slowly and prematurely—has to do with time, the seasons, and aging. On one hand, *parinama* is the natural rhythmic process of decay over time, the most inevitable part of aging and death. If you avoid peril long enough, you get old; then you die. On the other hand, parinama picks up pace when you miss the infinite opportunities to align yourself to the cosmic clock.

Through practice, we attune the body to the times and spaces of creation because without being in tune with them, we do not get very far. If you are not riding the time, you will live a mediocre life—probably a suffering life. Only if you are riding the time will you live an extraordinary life, which is what a human being and the human brain are designed for.[2]

Nature works in time through rhythms that can wipe your dis-ease slate clean. The 10 Habits of Body Thrive align you to the circadian, seasonal, and time-of-life rhythms. If you don't sync up with the macrocosmic rhythms, you tip the scale from ease to disease. In a nutshell, this is parinama.

Within time are cycles, and within cycles are junctures, which are like an anti-aging goldmine! When you take advantage of the daily, seasonal, and time-of-life junctures, you offload dis-ease. Through the 10 Habits of Body Thrive, you will attune to the rhythms and junctures inherent in time.

Inherent in ease is freedom, what the yogis call *svatantriya*. Ease comes through intentional habits that align you with flow. When you live into the 10 Habits of Body Thrive, you design an easeful and strong body, a clear and sharp mind, and dynamic relationships and become a vessel for spirit in action.

A Crash Course on Habit Evolution

When I studied Ayurveda, yoga, and enlightenment, my teachers told me which habits I should be doing daily. I didn't learn how to help myself and other humans to evolve their habits—that's the domain of behavioral science. Before learning the habits themselves, you will learn *how* to evolve your habits. As Mark Twain wrote, "Habit is habit, and not to be flung out of the window by any man, but coaxed downstairs a step at a time."

Empowered with a few specific tools for coaxing our habits along, we'll turn to Ayurveda to align our bodies and our lives into rhythm. When you know how to evolve your habits, progress happens with logic and is easy to leverage. We'll start with the most basic strategies and build from there. Refer to this chapter and pick a tactic when you want to evolve faster.

Identity Evolution and Your Hero's Journey

As Joseph Campbell would say, you are on your hero's journey. The call to adventure, the initiation, and the return with the elixir are the path of body thrive. The common theme on your hero's journey is that you can't remain the same. The initiation into better habits will change you. Your identity must uplevel. Habit and human potential expert James Clear explains: "The key to building lasting habits is focusing on creating a new identity first. Your current behaviors are simply a reflection of your current identity. What you do now is a mirror image of the type of person you believe that you are (either consciously or subconsciously). To change your behavior for good, you need to start believing new things about yourself."[1]

You can expect all the trials, exasperations, and pitfalls inherent in a hero's journey. Identify who you are becoming and who you have been, and the call to adventure will carry you through a rewarding return to a better version of yourself. Use the Identity-Evolving Worksheet in the free *Body Thrive Workbook*.

First, you need to get crystal clear on what *you* want. Be particular about your energy, your weight, your flexibility, your strength, and how your body ages. There is so much you can intentionally design. Check all that apply and add your own.

- Consistent energy
- Better sleep
- A toned, flexible body
- To wake rested, refreshed, clear-headed
- Smooth digestion
- Easy elimination
- To move easily
- Upbeat, relaxed emotions
- A more organized household
- Healthy, fast meal preparation
- Less stress, anxiety, or depression
- To age gracefully
- Healthy cravings
- More time

Circle what you want the most from what you checked above. This is your potential, and this book will get you on track to experiencing exactly the kind of integrated health called thrive. When you are thriving, you will also experience:

- A robust immune system
- Heartfelt, intimate relationships
- A clear purpose to your life
- An open and expansive perspective
- Fired-up dreams that you stretch for
- Getting body-smarter as you grow older
- Reinforcement that you are an inspiration and a help to others
- Speech that reflects your depth, your care, and connectivity

Check off any of those results you want and add your own. Get clear on exactly what you want. Unless you know your *what*, you'll miss the mark. Now, become even more clear about what you want in these three ways:

1. **Specific and measurable**   What you want needs to be specific and measurable. If it's a feeling, like less stress, you need to quantify it. Take a moment and get clear what this outcome will actually look like in real time. Less stress may turn into not working after dinner, being in bed by 10:00 p.m., hiring a housekeeper, setting an alarm for morning meditation, or cutting work back to a predetermined forty hours a week.

2. **Reality check**   Are you sure, with certainty, that you want that outcome? Do you need to tweak it? Remember, design with the end in mind.

3. **Timeline**   Put it on the clock. Your *what* has to be time-bound to a *when*. When is your desired completion date? Reverse engineer your future self.

Know Your Why

Now that you know your *what*, what is your *why*? Why do you want body thrive?

Your *why* needs to be laser sharp and one-pointed, what the yogis term *ekagrata*. Take a moment before proceeding. What is the *why* behind your desire for body thrive? Write that down. If my what is "I want to lose twelve pounds in ten weeks," my why is ". . . so that I have more energy for my kids, so that my clothes fit better, and so that it's easier to work out."

Get clear on your *why*, and it will serve as rocket fuel to move you through resistance. Resistance is the momentum of outdated patterns. Resistance can arise at any time in this process to pull you back to the starting line. When you are clear on your *why*, you have a rocket in your pocket.

Trust your *why*. Don't let the part of you that puts a kibosh on your potential get any face time here. Receive your intention like you would a gift from a wise elder who is looking out for you.

Use an Anchor Statement

An anchor statement grounds your big *why* by reducing it to a few words that center you. In yoga, the first anchor statements were termed *mahavakya* and have been used for millennia to anchor people's perspectives in their greatest capacities. Examples of mahavakyas:

- I am love itself.
- I am the same as the universe.
- All wisdom is available to me.

You can bring a mahavakya into your personal growing edge with an anchor statement:

- I am healthy, lean, and strong.
- I am grounded and steady.
- I rise and shine.
- I am energy in motion.
- I nourish myself.
- I choose contentment over stress.

Take a moment and turn your *why* into an anchor statement. Make it pithy, short, and reflective of the emotion you want to feel. You have decided. To paraphrase Paulo Coelho, whenever you make a decision, the whole universe conspires on your behalf. Write your *why* on a sticky note, and put it on your bathroom mirror. Each morning, it will form your intention, your *sankalpa*. Now you're using your high beams to get where you want to go while avoiding accidents along the way. When you don't know your *why*, you're myopic.

You have your mantra. Words crystalize into form. Speak them, and they become you. Prompt what you want to increase. William James, a nineteenth-century philosopher and psychologist, explained it this way:

> Seize the very first possible opportunity to act on every
> resolution you make, and on every emotional prompting
> you may experience in the direction of the habits you
> aspire to gain.[2]

By invoking the power of the word, you point your cellular vibration in the direction you want to go. When you do this repeatedly, you travel by a direct route. Use the worksheet called Your What, Your Why & Your Anchor in the free workbook at bodythrive.com/free.

Kaizen Your Habits

Kaizen means "good change" in Japanese, and it refers to the philosophy of applying continuous, daily, small improvements. Kaizen was developed in the United States during World War II (though it was not called by this name at the time) to efficiently convert and optimize factories for wartime production. Eventually, the kaizen method was adopted with remarkable success by leaders in personal development and habit evolution. We all know kaizen on some level; it's part of our ancestral folk medicine. Here are two:

- An apple a day keeps the doctor away.

- Early to bed, early to rise, makes a man healthy, wealthy, and wise.

Kaizen is the 1-percent improvement per day that leverages the compound effect. Look at the "Apple a day keeps the doctor away" example. Apples are chock-full of apple pectin, which has a nourishing, lubricating, and soothing effect on the colon. The pectin is a water-soluble fiber surrounded by a juicy fruit that makes a slippery goop. It winds through your guts and stimulates peristalsis. When taken daily, the apple promotes a lifetime of terrific bowel movements, which prevents the horrible diseases stemming from constipation and loose stools.

To accelerate your success with habit evolution, go black belt on kaizen. What is an easy upgrade—the smallest, most incremental improvement or baby step—you can make today that will make your tomorrow a little better, a little easier? Write that down and commit to it. The step or new habit should *underwhelm* you.

The problem with kaizen, for most of us, is that it seems too easy. When you get inspired to change or upgrade a habit, you want big returns. You bite off more than you can chew, which guarantees you'll fail. The kaizen approach makes the bite small enough that you hardly notice as it nudges you in the direction you want to go.

B. J. Fogg's Human Behavior Model

B. J. Fogg is the director of the Stanford Behavior Design Lab, where revolutions in behavior science are brewing. Fogg's breakthrough research on what makes us change behavior identifies that we need motivation, ability, and a trigger to converge in the same moment. Fogg's three-step method to better habits is:

1. **Get specific**   Translate target outcomes and goals into behaviors.

2. **Make it easy**   How can you make the behavior easy to do?

3. **Trigger the behavior**   What will prompt the behavior?[3]

To find your trigger for a better habit, use this simple sentence from Fogg: *"Right after I _____ , I will _____ ."*

Here are two examples: "Right after I wake up, I will scrape my tongue" or "Right after I do the dinner dishes, I will brush and floss." (You are less likely to eat before going to bed.)

Notice how simple and specific the behavior or new habit is. Double-check to make sure it's specific and easy. The idea is to set it low on the motivational scale. In the teeth-brushing example, you didn't say "Stop eating after washing dishes." You don't need motivation. You just need to set a trigger for a specific action. Fogg states that the best triggers are:

- location
- time
- emotional state
- other people
- an immediately preceding action

B. J. Fogg invites us to remember the secret to changing human behavior: keep both your desired behavior and your trigger simple. This means a lot from the dude with a PhD who runs the behavior lab at Stanford. As Fogg says, "Simplicity changes behavior."

Trigger, Habit, Reward

Another lesson from behavior science about automating habits worth familiarizing yourself with comes from Charles Duhigg, a journalist who reports on research about habits. In his bestselling book, *The Power of Habit*, Duhigg identifies three core elements that make up a habit loop:

1. A specific trigger or cue (remember Fogg's five common cues: location, time, emotional state, other people, immediately preceding action)

2. The routine or specific action

3. The reward or something that satisfies an urge[4]

Duhigg forewarns that redesigning your habits is a bit of a process. Figuring out your current undesired behaviors in terms of the actual cues and rewards requires sleuthing. When redesigning habits, you need to identify the current cue that is signaling the outdated habit and corresponding reward. But before that, you need to find a more appropriate reward.

"By experimenting with different rewards, you can isolate what you are *actually* craving, which is essential in redesigning the habit," explains Duhigg. Once that is solved, you figure out your cue and make a better plan. He gives a framework for the process:

1. Identify the routine.

2. Experiment with rewards.

3. Isolate the cue.

4. Have a plan.

You can see the overlap in Duhigg's and Fogg's research and conclusions. Make a habit go from automated unconscious to conscious. Notice your habits. Start with checking out what is going on in slow motion in your decision-making. Identify the habit. As you get fancier and more advanced, notice the habit trigger or cue. To check it out, slow down what's happening when you act on a habit you do or don't want. Make your triggers or routines go from unconscious to conscious. Once you've observed that, make a better plan.

B. J. Fogg is the father of "tiny habits." He believes that the plan should be a tiny plan. You could think of your tiny plan—your kaizen iterations—as a series of small, doable experiments. This way you get more data, and that feedback will inform your behavior via your next plan or small experiment.

Habit evolution becomes fun when we consciously design our habits via habit triggers and rewards.

"Yes, And"

The "yes, and" idea comes from a rule of improvisational comedy that requires members of a troop to say "yes" to whatever invitation they have been given and then to add to the building narrative. "Yes, and" is the opposite of "no, but." The rule is similar to a yogic principle of seeing the *shri*, or recognizing the good, the true, or the beautiful in any given situation.

As you read through your habits, the voice in your head will naturally resist some habit changes. The voice may say, "No, but I can't do that. I can't go to bed any earlier. I have so much that needs to get done." That is a classic "no, but."

See if you can turn your "no, buts" into "yes, ands": "Yes, getting more sleep sounds great. And I can probably go to bed five minutes earlier this week." For those responsible for children, teach them about "no, buts" and "yes, ands." You can make it a game with yourself and those with whom your habits intertwine.

Architect Your Choices, Design Your Environment

You want to make your new pattern the default. You want to make your old pattern more difficult to reinstate. Set up your outer environment to encourage the budding habit. "Choice architecture" is the careful design of the environments in which you make choices. Your environment is malleable, so your home should continually shift as a reflection of your upgrading habits. Essentially, you want to make it hard to slip into habits you don't want to reinforce. At the same time, make habits you *do* want to reinforce easier to do. Here are some examples of how to architect your environment to stabilize budding habits:

- If you want to eat healthfully, stock your fridge with cut-up, ready-to-eat vegetables. Compost or give away any processed food.

- If you want to start jogging in the morning, set out your running outfit and shoes the night before.

- If you want to start drinking herbal tea instead of coffee, set out your teapot and tea bag the night before. If you can't bear to part with your coffee, put it in the garage. That way, during the time you walk out to fetch it, you have the opportunity to reflect about whether you *truly* want coffee. On the way to the garage, you might change your mind and opt to drink the tea instead.

- If you want to start meditating, create a space to sit, and then practice sitting there for just a minute at a time. Set up this area so it invites you to sit quietly.

- If you want more space and time in your life, declutter your house once and for all with Marie Kondo's method, made famous in her best-seller, *The Life-Changing Magic of Tidying Up*. Your possessions influence your habits. If you have too much stuff, it's easy to become trapped in outdated habits. But refining your environment allows you the space to become who you want to be next. Kondo's book shows you how to clean out your living area and purge everything from your wardrobe, book collection, file cabinets, and kitchen-tool collection—right down to your last paperclip. In my next book, *Awake Living*, I dive deep into how to architect your home and space to attune to your dharma, or purposeful life.

If your home environment creates barriers to your new habit, you will fail. Design your space to help you gain traction. Write down ten ideas for ways you can design your environment to make your new habits happen. Then take action.

Work toward Habit Automation

At some point in your Body Thrive journey, you'll become aware that the habits you longed to establish have become routine. You do them efficiently, without resistance, without deciding in the moment.

Making too many decisions creates decision fatigue. The beauty of habit automation is that you only decide once. You decide, "I will eat dinner by 6:00 p.m." You decide on your trigger. Now the work becomes a daily rhythm.

When good habits are your automatic default, you free up tremendous energy for creativity. Work toward an automatic daily rhythm, and you'll smooth the edgy path of habit evolution.

Power of the Posse

Our peers can elevate or undermine us. In this process of upleveling your habits, you want to choose your peer support wisely. Connect with people who are on the wavelength you want to be on. For me, that took consciously putting myself in groups (like the online Body Thrive group), hiring coaches, and attending trainings. You can put together a local *Body Thrive* book group (see the guide at the back of the book) and plunge in together.

If at any time in the process of evolving your habits you feel stuck or overwhelmed, chances are you need the power of the posse. Otherwise, you'll feel frustrated and overwhelmed by the "running in place" conversations. When you try to evolve in isolation or against the momentum of your current company, you make it ten times harder.

I place myself in specific situations—like coaching groups and training events—where I'm bound to meet people who inspire me. We become fast friends and intentionally look for ways to support each other. I like how investor guru Warren Buffett describes this basic teaching: "It's better to hang out with people better than you. Pick out associates whose behavior is better than yours, and you'll drift in that direction."[5] You may find your growth path is more in sync with new friends than folks you have known your whole life.

Discover Your Keystone

For those who aren't masons or architecture aficionados, the *keystone* is the stone in the top of an archway. The keystone enables the arch to bear the weight of the load above, which may include the roof or another story. It is the rock that bears the most weight, keeping the archway from collapsing.

Your keystone habit is the habit that when you do it, you automatically connect to some of the other habits. Your keystone habit builds tensile strength across your other habits. It also stands the strongest on its own. If you could choose only one habit on a given day, this would be the one you'd choose because you get the most bang for your habit buck. In the journey ahead, you want to zone in on the habit that holds together the universe of you, at the level where you can bear the load of life. What is the key habit that allows you to be a better version of yourself?

My keystone habit is to eat an earlier, lighter dinner. If I eat an earlier, lighter dinner, I get tired earlier. I get a great night's sleep, ergo I wake up early with plenty of time to myself. I meditate and work out before the day officially begins. Throughout the day, because my body is oxygenated, my mind is centered, and I crave healthy food.

An earlier, lighter dinner is the keystone that holds my Body Thrive routine together. If I blow that habit, the next day is a risky, uncertain matter—aka a crapshoot. If I make this habit a priority, I can uphold mountains on a regular basis. As you move through the habits, use the Keystone Habit Worksheet in the workbook.

Part 2

The 10 Habits of Body Thrive

HABIT 1

Eat an Earlier, Lighter Dinner

WHAT TO DO

Eat your last meal of the day by 6:00 or 7:00 p.m., or at least three hours before bed. For dinner, choose soups and salads over solid foods, because food with more water content is easier to digest. Eat more green and nonstarchy root vegetables and fewer grains, legumes, meat, and dairy. After dinner, close your kitchen and don't snack.

WHY YOU WANT TO DO IT

Dinner should be supplemental—a little extra—not the main event. You will wake up feeling lighter and energized the next day when you keep dinner supplemental. You'll make your body's job easier. You'll have fewer aches and pains as you age, and you won't get fat, tired, and overwhelmed. That's a big payoff for a small meal.

HOW TO START

Eat a respectable lunch, which must include protein and fat, even dessert if you want it. Wind back your last meal of the day fifteen minutes earlier until you're eating by 6:00 p.m. Reverse-engineer your schedule to make it happen. If you eat dessert, have it immediately following dinner, then brush and floss your teeth. Works like a charm.

"I didn't care about the weight. My body can carry extra weight, and it didn't seem like a big deal. My issue was about my integrity. I'd wake up tired and groggy," explained Ginger, one of the many Body Thrive members I've coached. "Now I wake up clear and light and bright. My body is happier. That's why I eat an earlier, lighter dinner."

Ginger had wanted to eat an earlier, lighter dinner, but couldn't figure out how it could work. Her kids didn't get home until 6:45 p.m., and the family didn't eat dinner until 7:00 or 7:30. She was operating under the outdated belief that if she didn't eat with her family at the evening meal, she was an inadequate mother.

This belief may sound silly or sane to you. It doesn't matter. What matters is that Ginger's belief created a blockade between how she felt in her body and how she *wanted* to feel in her body.

I asked Ginger to experiment. From experience in coaching clients through detoxes, I've found that inviting people to run experiments with their diet and habits leads to a perspective of curiosity. *What helps me thrive?* That's the question.

I asked Ginger when she would like to eat dinner if she didn't have family obligations and what she would eat. After feeling into her body and allowing herself the freedom to dream big for herself, Ginger replied: "I come home from work at 5:00 p.m. If I were alone, I would do two to fifteen minutes of meditation or deep breathing, and then prepare a simple dinner for myself." Once she knew what *she* wanted, she could work her family responsibilities around her needs, instead of the other way around. She reversed the order of her evening obligations to fit her long-term goals.

Ginger knew this change was a big deal. The family dinner was an old pattern, instilled by her mother and grandmother. When a pattern carries ancestral weight, it feels more like concrete than moldable clay. I invited Ginger to talk to her family about her needs and her desire to eat earlier, by herself, and to enjoy a cup of herbal tea while they ate later. We both knew this would be a monumental shift for her and her family.

Ginger decided to use a time trigger (coming home from work) to inject the updated behavior. She committed to injecting conscious breath work for two to fifteen minutes immediately when she got home. Being a yoga student, Ginger knew that a few minutes of conscious breath work would shift her brain chemistry from reactive mode into proactive mode—from stress to ease—even if she started with just two minutes. A calmer, more centered experience would pave the way to making better choices around when and what to eat. Ginger's new sequence went like this:

1. Return home from work; set down her bag; wash her face, hands, and feet; and go directly to her meditation cushion.

2. Play an audio instruction for breath work from her smartphone.

3. With mind clear and body refreshed, prepare a quick, lovely, light meal for herself.

4. Sit down and eat in silence, enjoying the time by herself.

5. Feeling nourished and relaxed, finish preparing an evening meal for her family.

6. Sit, drink tea, and be with her family during the evening meal.

Ginger found that she no longer minded popping out of her chair for family requests, which tend to arise during the evening meal, though this used to aggravate her when she was trying to nourish herself at the same time. Did her family mind that she was sipping tea when they were eating? No. "My kids adapted," she said. "Sure, at first it was weird, but we all got used to it after a week. Now I know the consequences of my habits on every aspect of my life. How I feel now is all the impetus I need to maintain my momentum on this new path."

Such is the power of the earlier, lighter dinner. Over time, she knew she might sway her family's schedule toward an earlier, lighter dinner; however, before inviting them to change, she took the power of her body back into her own hands. She changed her behavior and changed her results by changing the order of her evening routine. Let's see why this habit worked wonders for Ginger.

Order Matters

The order of *what* you do *when* is called *krama*, the sequence that allows consciousness and energy to flow for optimal health. Any effective yoga teacher has had weeks of training on sequencing or ordering poses to achieve a desired result: opening the body's subtle channels into flow and strengthening those channels for more capacity, vibrancy, and higher consciousness. Likewise, any computer coder knows how to sequence the right symbols to get the desired results.

When you're not getting the results you're after in your life, investigate what you're doing and in what order you're doing it. If you have the right inputs, but the wrong order, you won't get what you're after.

Let's apply this to food. If you eat nutrient-rich food at the wrong time of day, your body can't digest the nutrients. The night before you want to have a great day in body, mind, and spirit, eat an earlier, lighter dinner.

The order in which you do the same things day in and day out determines who you become. If you regularly eat a heavier dinner and try to wake early to exercise or do yoga, your practice won't progress. Your body would rather be inert like a cat after feasting on a mouse. If you hit your mat on an empty stomach or after a pint of fresh green juice, your body may be very happy to twist, bend, and go upside down.

Order is crucial. Start the night *before* the day you want to feel like a million bucks. Mess with the krama of the night before and you enter the land of inefficiency. When you get the order wrong, it's like rolling a boulder up a mountain: more energy is expended and nothing more is gained. Something is lost.

Akrama, or going against the rhythm, reminds me of the fourth circle of Dante's *Inferno*. Men who squandered money (or energy) pushed big boulders around, going nowhere forever. Energy amassed, energy expended, nothing gained. When you eat heavily at night, you generate more work for your body and you misuse your body's resources.

I know this firsthand. The first half of my life I ate a heavier, later dinner. I grew up in suburban Massachusetts. My dad, bless him, commuted twenty miles through traffic to Cambridge five days a week. When he returned home, usually ten to eleven hours after he'd left, he enjoyed kicking off his shoes and having my sister or me pour him a stiff drink.

For my siblings and me, the wait was excruciating. We were student athletes. We would wait until after 7:00 p.m. for dinner, our most nutrient-dense meal. By this time, our blood sugar had crashed, and we were exhausted. We had passed the stage where our bodies could digest heavy food. Our digestion was shutting down for the night, not gearing up.

A pattern set in motion stays in motion. I inadvertently continued this late dinner pattern into my midtwenties and then spent a few years aligning my mealtimes with what I was learning from Ayurveda and yoga. Late dinners lead to staying up later to digest and getting a lethargic morning start. If your schedule is inefficient for your body, you'll always feel behind. You'll feel like you're perpetually trying to keep up—that there isn't enough time in your day for what you need to do. Let's dive into why.

Agni and *Ama*

Ayurveda is brilliant in its obsession with the power of digestion—the fire, the bile, the enzymes that convert food into energy and body. The capacity that governs metabolism, digestion, absorption, and assimilation is named *agni*. Turning food into energy and bodily tissue is agni's job.

Agni has its own krama within the twenty-four-hour day, warming up by midmorning, blazing at midday, and setting with the sun.

Turning heavy food into energy and bodily tissue after the sun goes down is recklessly taxing for your physiology. The outer ecosystem and your inner ecosystem respond to the natural law of "like increases like." It's easy to forget that human physiology, including the design of the human digestive tract, evolved over millennia, shaped by the natural laws here on Earth.

Homo sapiens is a diurnal species, unlike our cat or dog. Historically, we ate during the day, when we could see. Our eyes can see more vibrant colors than Fluffy's, whose eyes are designed for low light and night vision. Fluffy doesn't care if he can see the mouse as he bites off the head. We like to see what we're eating.

Our bile cycle is optimized to digest the best between 10:00 a.m. and 2:00 p.m., when sunlight makes our world appear in Technicolor. When you eat a good meal around this time, you have the rest of the day to digest and use the energy from your food. If you eat most of your nutrients or calories later in the day, you make agni's job difficult by eating at a time of day when your digestion would rather chill out than get fired up. Eating too much too late challenges your digestion. When done habitually, undigested food builds in your gut. Energetically this degenerative habit depresses your physiology as an entire system. When you subject the universe of you to heavy, late-evening dinners as you age, you'll degenerate. For me even as a child, the consequences of large, late dinners were headaches, snot-filled sinuses, a heavier body weight, and lower body integrity (or body-based self-esteem).

The sections of your gut should alternate between dynamic and restful—when the stomach is finished, it should be resting while the small intestine is working, and so on. If your gut is healthy and in rhythm, you deeply digest your nutrients. Deep nutrification fuels your mind and energy body and regenerates your bodily tissue. When agni is strong and balanced, you feel satiated and relaxed after eating, and vibrant between long stretches between meals, or long stretches between the last meal of the day and the breaking of the fast the next day. You may have heard of the long stretches of digestive rest called *intermittent fasting* or *intermittent nourishment*. Your digestive process likes to work and rest. In Chinese medicine our digestive apparatus is considered "masculine": it works, then rests. The lungs and heart are "feminine": they are steady, constant rhythm. When you align with your agni, your digestion and your energy become smooth and easy. No bloat, no gas, no constipation, no snot the next day.

The word for "undigested" is *ama* in Sanskrit. It is the dirt in the grease of your engine, the gum in the works. Ama is the gunky residue left over from poorly digested food. Ama leads to energy inefficiency, which leads to disease. When you eat asynchronously, or akrama, you disrupt the rhythm of your digestive tract. If the heavy dinner becomes repetitive, the ama moves from the gut into the blood and the joints, rendering the body lethargic and stiff in the morning.

The next day you feel the sludge in your system, the junk in your trunk, and the pessimism in your attitude. The stress leads to inflammation. Add the compound effect to this pattern, and you end up with chronic inflammation. No fun. If this is you, know that you can change your reality and wake up with more ease, energy, and flexibility in about a week's time.

The solution is simple. Line up *when* you eat with your human agni cycle. Agni is strongest in the middle of the day. Adjust your schedule to eat your most nutrient-loaded sustaining meal when the sun is bright in the sky.

We used to know this. The midday meal, formerly known as "dinner," was shoved to late in the day with the transition from farm to factory. The recent lunch-dinner combo invention is evidently epidemically dangerous for our health.

Back in the day, supper was soup. "Sup" and "sip" both mean to take liquid food. Farmers would have a pot of soup on the stove all day, and in the early evening, they would "sup" the soup at supper. Today the evening meal is showtime as far as the three meals go. Inspect photos of people fifty years ago with their lithe, strong bodies, and you find it's worth a deeper investigation into our newfangled eating cycles in the age of big lunches and big dinners.

Make Space to Keep Pace

Your stomach is designed to become full and empty, like a gas tank. But unlike a gas tank, your stomach expands and contracts. If you don't actively engage the contraction part of the cycle with daily fasting before breakfast, then you're unintentionally creating an endless expansion cycle. Just check the recent statistics on how Americans' waistlines are expanding: the *average* waist circumference is forty inches for men and thirty-eight for women,[1] and almost 40 percent of US adults in 2015–2016 were considered obese.[2]

As a culture, we're stuffed. We're expanding and not contracting. We're not allowing the rest phase of the digestive cycle. This is equivalent to rapid inhales and short exhales. A slow contraction part of the breath cycle creates rest, renewal, and room for the next inhale to be received. If the pulsation is too fast, you hyperventilate.

Digestion works the same way. The long exhale part of the cycle is when the stomach is empty. Allow your body a fast between dinner and breakfast. Thirteen hours is your goal. Dinner by 6:00 p.m., bed by 9:30, breakfast between 7:00 and 8:00 a.m., lunch around noon. No snacking. Deep rest and internal healing require space in your belly. Are you a lead belly or a light belly before bed?

Good digestion needs gravity.[3] We're centered on a north-south axis. Lying down with a heavy stomach feels horrible because you are on the wrong axis. Plus, your breath won't be as deep and easy all night long. With a bloated belly, the inhale is shallow, which triggers the nervous system into a stress response. Shallow breathing puts your body in a stress cycle.[4] If you go to bed on a full belly, you'll wake up with less oxygen in your blood and less life-force energy, what the yogis call *prana*, in your cells.

What If Early Is Impossible?

After a decade of clinical work as an Ayurvedic practitioner, I've heard a plethora of legitimate reasons why it's not possible to eat an earlier, lighter dinner. Most of them sound reasonable:

- A big lunch makes me sleepy.

- My kids don't get home from sports until 7:00 p.m.

- It takes time to make a nice dinner, so we eat at 8:00 p.m.

- I take or teach a yoga or fitness class after 7:00 p.m.

- My husband and I like to eat after working out. It's the only time of the day we can connect.

Many of us eat later, heavier dinners out of social habit. We were raised to value the evening meal as the quintessential family time. Yet, as a culture, we now have epidemic issues with mood (anxiety and depression), inadequate sleep, and more-than-adequate body weight. Our cultural habits violate our bodies' most basic needs. From a biological perspective, the later, heavier dinner is an early, slow, dramatic death sentence.

The ancient authoritative text on Ayurveda, the *Charaka Samhita*, says that when "the agni of an individual is balanced, or *sama agni*, then health, happiness, and longevity are a natural effect. But if the agni of a person is vitiated, the disturbed metabolism engenders ill health and disease. Hence, agni is said to be the base (*mool*) of life."[5]

Given that agni is the root of your health, you may want to adjust your schedule to eat "dinner" at lunch and sup on soup or salad later in the day.

What's for Dinner?

If you've had a good lunch, soup and/or salad is all you need for an evening meal. Soups and salads are quick to prepare and easy to digest due to their high water and vegetable content. In salads and soups, the different foods or plants combine before they enter your body, requiring less energy for digestion.

Most dinners at my house take less than twenty minutes to prepare and about twenty minutes to eat. I call dinner "the biggest non-event" in my household. Our soups and salads focus on vegetables from our yard or regional farms. Because dinner doesn't take much energy to digest, we are energized afterward to have fun and burn a few calories before bed to boot.

Rather than preparing and eating an elaborate meal after work that my gut can't digest gracefully, I'd rather spend time playing, taking care of household tasks, or relaxing with my peeps. We stroll together, ride bikes around the neighborhood, or rally for housework or yardwork.

Light movement after an evening meal feels great, aids digestion, and helps our systems drop into evening chill-out mode. Our exception to this rule is Sunday dinner. About once per week, I prepare an elaborate meal. We dine and relax, enjoying each other's company. We clean up and are done by 5:00 p.m. Here are some menu items:

- Miso soup and green salad with fresh veggies and ginger-miso dressing

- French onion soup with local artisan bread

- Vegetarian chili

- Greek salad

- Minestrone soup

- Green salad with potatoes and green beans

- Carrot coconut-curry soup and avocado on rice cakes

- Tostadas with avocado and sauerkraut (great for travel)

- Raw tomato soup

- Spicy lentil soup with crème fraîche

- Salad Niçoise

- Roasted sweet potatoes, brussels sprouts, and parmesan

- Asian cabbage salad

- Arugula with roasted beets and goat cheese

- Kimchi and sweet-and-sour soup

Soup and/or salad—you get the picture. You want dinner to be simple to prepare and simple to digest. If you don't like to cook, eat out for lunch. That way you'll be satisfied with a simple green salad or soup for dinner. Learn how to make a few easy soups, and you'll be all set. See the workbook at bodythrive.com/free for simple soup recipes.

Weekly Meal Planner

When changing habits, it's normal to have times of high and low motivation. Perhaps right now you're inspired. You're stoked. You're highly motivated. You want results, and you're ready for action. Take that motivation and make a food plan.

The Weekly Meal Planner is a blank chart that will help you plan what you're eating this week. (You'll find it in the downloadable *Body Thrive Workbook*, bodythrive.com/free.) Use your Weekly Meal Planner to set your *sankalpa*, your intention with food. Planning paves the way for aligned action.

With any habit change, get specific and put it on a timeline or on your calendar. Schedule an hour to get organized with your food plan. When that hour arrives, start with the nine steps to weekly meal planning:

1. Print four copies of the Weekly Meal Planner. Put blanks in a snazzy folder to store in your kitchen, perhaps with your recipe books. Store used meal planners in your folder to reuse later.

2. Check your cupboards, your fridge, your garden, and anywhere else you store food. Notice what you already have.

3. Take out a few recipe books that seem to jump off your shelf, or open your laptop to your favorite search engine. Google your diet preferences, such as Ayurveda, paleo, raw, vegan, locavore, or whatever describes the foods you want to make. Create a folder just for recipes in your search engine's bookmarks.

4. Get out your calendar. Your daily food prep needs to fit into your preexisting day, or you need to adjust your calendar.

5. Fill in your Weekly Meal Planner for this week. Underwhelm yourself. Make it easy to prepare. If you eat out, write in what you intend to order to keep in alignment with the body you want. You can even verbally rehearse your order.

6. Update your calendar. Schedule your daily food prep times with specific actions. Then schedule when you'll grocery shop or harvest.

7. Write your grocery shopping list.

8. Pin your Meal Planner to your fridge. If your fridge is cluttered, declutter it. Make space to keep pace.

9. Check your plan daily.

Like any new habit, it's a much bigger deal in the beginning but effortless once automated. You can become an expert at streamlining food prep. See the "Kitchen Sadhana" chapter on page 213 for ideas.

Get Specific and Repetitive

If you're changing *when* you are eating, identify a time trigger and a specific habit change. For instance, my client Ginger used the "five o'clock get home from work" time trigger to start a new habit of meditation. That was enough to set an earlier, lighter dinner in motion.

If you're changing *what* you eat, use the nine-step weekly meal plan on page 43. Once Ginger dialed in when she ate, she wanted to diversify what she ate. Desiring more seasonal and local foods, she took the time to plan, shop, and prep.

Don't get fancy. If you get fancy, you'll fail. Pick only one to two new recipes per week. Eat slight variations on the same thing for lunch and dinner. This saves time, money, and digestive energy. You may think it sounds boring to have the same thing for lunch and dinner. Maybe it is, but that mild repetition frees up the rest of your life to be far more exciting than time in the kitchen or time with indigestion.

Baby Steps

Did you know we lose weight when we eat from smaller plates? Inspect dinnerware from fifty years ago, and you'll find the plates are one-third smaller. A recent study replaced twelve-inch plates with ten-inch plates. People ate 22 percent fewer calories.[6] No willpower required.

Start with where you are, and take baby steps to where you want to be. Ginger's transformation occurred when she took what she wanted—to feel better in the morning—and broke it down into small, doable, reasonable actions. She started with two minutes of breath work upon arriving home after work.

Identify steps that seem doable and failproof with all you have going on in your life right now. You don't need to move up your meal-time by an hour and a half. You don't need to cancel date night. You don't need to exclusively eat soups, salads, and sauerkrauts ad infinitum. That would only trigger your inner rebel into rebellion. You don't need to set strict rules or regulations for your behavior. Creating unnecessary tension will only undermine your thrive. If you are a rebel or rule breaker, you'll only break your own rules anyway. If you are a goody-two-shoes, you'll only disappoint yourself when you can't live up to your rules, and that will trigger your pattern of psychosomatic self-flagellation. Start with a specific behavior change that seems easy but will be effective enough to notice if it's working over time. At the end of this chapter are tips on where to begin.

Remember, you are more interested in small gains than a perfect picture. Praise your progress. Repeat your anchor statement. Notice the difference and be carried by your nascent momentum. Undesirable habits fall away naturally like dead leaves off autumn trees. Earlier, lighter dinners are not about becoming antisocial or dogmatic; they're about slow, steady changes that support your physiology. Surprisingly, your social schedule will adjust. And you never know: this just might be the keystone habit that unlocks the door to your body thrive.

Reverse-Engineer Your Success

Often there's too big a gap between how your life is now and how you want it to be. The gap may seem impossible to leap—so don't. Simply build a bridge backward from where you want to be. If other people are involved, the chapter called How to Evolve Your Habits in Relationships on page 115 will be essential to your progress. For now, start with one small change you can make right off the bat, all by yourself: to eat either a little earlier or a little lighter at night. Write down that change right now and put it in your calendar, repetitively. Like the saying goes, "What gets scheduled gets done."

Over the years, I've worked with dozens of yoga teachers who taught in the evenings. As they studied Ayurveda with me, they began to resent nights away from home. Their pattern was dinner after class—after 9:00 p.m.—which pushed back bedtime, making waking early for meditation and personal practice not fun. They wanted to live the teachings, but changing evening to morning classes wasn't an option in the short term.

Applying the one small change principle, I invited the teachers to eat a light dinner before class. Many were having a snack then anyway. Adding half an avocado to their snack before class and a cup of broth, miso soup, or herbal tea with milk after class was often all it took for them to make it until breakfast without true hunger on teaching nights. The warm beverage before bed engenders the feeling of nourishment without weighing you down. Another option is to switch from three meals a day to two—at around 10:00 a.m. and 4:00 p.m.

My mom used the phrase "kitchen closed" to signify when we were not allowed to graze through the fridge or cupboards. We ate real meals. After meals, the kitchen was closed. My students embed this mantra to train themselves to stop eating after dinner. The handful of roasted grapes or piece of chocolate puts digestion into overtime. Like the example with the breath, you're not allowing the exhale before the next inhale when you eat at night.

If you eat dessert, make it a light reward for cleaning up, then close your kitchen. If you live with others, close the kitchen to yourself by brushing and flossing immediately after your last meal of the day.

Troubleshooting Night Jobs

Many people don't have the gorgeous luxury of sleeping at night and working during the day, including nurses, doctors, cops, security guards, chefs, bartenders, servers, musicians, and many others.

The problem is that working nights over time wreaks serious havoc on the universe of you. You need to dial in habits that support your body in these contrary conditions. If you wait tables four nights a week or work the night shift at the hospital two nights a week, you need to make the most of the nights you have at home. You need a very strong immune system to work nights consistently.

On one hand, you're moving against the massive momentum of circadian rhythm; on the other hand, as a species we are amazingly resilient. To work nights *and* cultivate your immune system, you need rhythms that nourish your body. On your nights off, protect those evenings as if your life force depends on it, because it does. Create quiet evenings at home and wind down early—even if you're in your twenties and want to party like a rock star. Prioritize your bigger picture. Sure, party once every week or two. The other nights, stay home. Go to bed early. Wake up early and plug your attention into your long-term vision.

On nights you work, eat as early as you can in the evening; that will tide you over until bedtime. Eat whole foods and nourishing fats to stabilize your blood sugar. When you get home in the wee hours, have a cup of herbal tea with licorice root and fennel seeds. Rub some lavender or cedarwood essential oil on your feet and hit the sack. Don't eat late at night or before bed. Streamline your wind-down routine to be quick and efficient (as per the routines in the next chapter).

If you're working nights and need stimulants like caffeine or refined sugars for energy, you're digging into visceral adulteration. Your skin will age quickly. You'll feel uncentered, and it will become more challenging to step into your dreams. Do a short detox to decrease your need for stimulants. Your body has a tough enough job as it is, living in an inverse cycle. Get clean to dig a deep, authentic wellspring of energy.

If you already have poor immunity and poor energy, or if you feel stuck in an off-cycle in your life, start to plan ahead for what you want your daily routines to look like in the future. Spend some time each week cultivating a plan B or exit strategy to fit your body's desired rest rhythm.

Are You Stuffed or Content?

As you work and rework this habit of eating light, early dinners, use the following assessment to see if you need to take this habit seriously:

- You feel great with your weight.

- You wake up feeling light and energized.

- After dinner you act on the desire to move, take a walk, do household tasks, or play outside.

- After dinner you don't feel stuffed; you feel content.

- You feel a natural fatigue, but not exhaustion, at the end of the day.

- When you go to bed, your belly feels empty and light, but you're not hungry.

These signs indicate your dinner is light and early enough. Once you have these earlier, lighter dinners in motion, you've set the stage for the next two habits, which involve times for going to bed and waking up. So really, you get three habits dialed in for the effort of one.

TIPS FOR EATING AN EARLIER, LIGHTER DINNER

- "Sup" your soup or salad—keep it a one-pot meal.

- Use a bowl or ten-inch plate.

- Use the Weekly Meal Planner worksheet.

- Get organized with your grocery shopping.

- Be repetitive with lunch and dinner if you don't have much time to make food.

- Eat your local and seasonal crops in abundance.

- Prep your dinner when you prep your breakfast.

- Bake root vegetables in the morning and reheat them in the evening.

- Use a slow cooker.

- Plan ahead.

- Try two minutes of slow, deep breathing before walking into the kitchen.

HABIT 2

Go to Bed Early

WHAT TO DO

Enhance your bedtime routine with nourishing habits
that wind you down. Land yourself in bed with lights
out by 10:00 p.m. If you have fatigue, dis-ease, or
immune issues and your nerves need more juice, aim
for a 9:00 p.m. bedtime. Wind your bedtime routine
back by fifteen minutes per week, or an hour per month,
until you get there. Even night owls thrive when they
become morning doves.

WHY YOU WANT TO DO IT

Energetically, you want to start most of your tomorrows
on a full tank of gas. If you go to bed after 10:00 p.m.,
you're spending tomorrow's fuel today—meaning you're
running a deficit. By going to bed earlier, you can rise
earlier and witness the glory of dawn, bright-eyed and
bushy-tailed. Would you rather play your A game—or
just try to keep up?

HOW TO START

Reverse-engineer a bedtime fifteen minutes earlier in your schedule until you end up consistently well-rested. Use your phone timer to alert you when to kick-start your unplug, unwind, and into-the-sack routine. Your reward at the end of a day well lived is an effective, feel-good, wind-down routine and well-deserved rest. When you hit the sack, relax your body and feel the sensations of physical and mental fatigue or agitation. Release. Unfurl. Welcome restoration and rest.

Our grandmothers were raised on this basic body wisdom: "Early to bed, early to rise, makes a man healthy, wealthy, and wise." Chances are, if you are statistically average, you may act like you're exempt. What is the price of not heeding your body's fundamental restoration cycle?

As a culture, we have no idea how tired we really are. Our fatigue is ingrained into the fabric of our physiology, and it slowly wreaks havoc on our immunity. Your immune system's job is to keep the universe of you together, integrated, grounded, and strong. When you get honest with your cultural overstimulation and overwhelm, which leads to your personal fatigue, you notice just how deep you've fallen into the inadequate sleep pit of despair. More often than not, you're in over your head.

In our modern times, we have the coolest high-tech connection devices, but our body's connection device—our protection or immune system—is shredded. Autoimmune diseases are increasing, and more are being identified. I bet you know five people with one of the following diseases of broken-down immune function:

- Rheumatoid arthritis
- Hashimoto's thyroiditis
- Type 1 diabetes
- Multiple sclerosis

- Graves' disease
- Lupus
- Fibromyalgia
- Psoriasis
- Inflammatory bowel disease

The autoimmune list now includes over eighty diseases. Not good. Plus, the Asthma and Allergy Foundation of America estimates that each year more than 50 million Americans experience allergies—a less severe manifestation of an aberrant immune response—and that allergies are the sixth leading cause of chronic illness in the United States.[1] When we talk about the immune system, we are also talking about body integrity, the state of being whole and undivided. When you have immune integrity, you're strong within yourself against disease. You are your own united front. When you're repeatedly tired, your inner troops lose connection and identity, and fall apart.

Most kids and teens are tired. Most adults are exhausted. The US Centers for Disease Control (CDC) reports that insufficient sleep is a public health epidemic.[2] (*Epidemic* means a widespread occurrence of a disease in a community.) Overall, sleep duration appears to have decreased by 1.5 to 2 hours per night (around 25 percent) during the second half of the twentieth century.[3] As a culture, we're out of sync with energy integrity, which disrupts our immune function.

Your sleep cycle is synchronized by the day-night or light-dark rhythms outside your body. When you align with circadian rhythm, health ensues. When you develop abnormal circadian rhythms, you risk obesity, diabetes, depression, bipolar disorder, and seasonal affective disorder, to name a few proven problems.[4] When you don't get enough sleep, you are also more likely to become a host for cancer.[5] When you're playing with electrical gadgets or looking at a screen after 10:00 p.m., you're playing with fire.

Deep, consistent sleep after dusk until before the dawn is the nectar of your immune function. If you burn the midnight oil consistently, you burn yourself out. The way Ayurveda explains it is that the dominant energy between 10:00 p.m. and 2:00 a.m. is governed by the subtle metabolic energy of *pitta*, which is the energy of digestion, metabolism, and detoxification. (See the illustration on page 55.) If you're not in bed early enough, your body won't detoxify the day's buildup of mental and physical stresses.

The hours before 10:00 p.m. belong to the slow, anabolic, replenishing energy of *kapha*, the energy of connection or cohesion, which engenders contentment and relaxation. When you fall asleep before 10:00, you get replenished by the calm, soothing recalibration of kapha. The energy you fall asleep in becomes the dominant energy in your sleep cycle.

This mellow, reflective energy of early evening builds and renews. If you're attuned to the kapha nature of this time of day, you'll notice that the vibe is sweet, the conversation easy and fluid. You'll be in the reflective aspect of the cycle of consciousness, reviewing your day and your life. Attunement becomes atonement. The atmosphere becomes more dense; your eyelids get heavy. If you are in sync, you know it's time for bed.

When you stay up after 10:00 p.m., you aggravate your inner housekeeping systems, which need good sleep to function. If you're a night owl, you make it harder for your body to clean house. Over time, this overwhelms your immune system. In Ayurveda, we call worn-down immune function "low *ojas*."

Night Owls: Beware the Evil Second Wind

As the day comes to a close, you may be accustomed to overriding your body's quietening messages. If you were raised in a household of night owls who disregarded the circadian wind-down—that slow, drowsy, cosmic, anabolic, kapha shift in energy—you may not know it exists. Yet, if you've ever gone camping, you can tap into this feeling. When the sun goes down, you get drowsy and go to bed earlier. Have you noticed that without electric lights you can feel your sleepiness?

Many parents of younger children create the feeling when they dim the lights to read bedtime stories. Through winding down their kids, they feel their own fatigue. Now compare this to when you fire up the tube or tablet after dinner. Ever notice that you felt tired when you started your screen time, but before you know it, you get a second wind?

That is the *evil* second wind. If you'd gone to bed early, you'd have been asleep for it. This rising energy is supposed to clean your inner body-house while you dream-travel the waves of the etheric realm. But if you press "next episode" on your remote or open the next email, your mind and spirit take in yet more information instead of processing the day you just lived. This is the equivalent of helping yourself to seconds when you are already full. Mental digestion and reflection are key to building ojas.

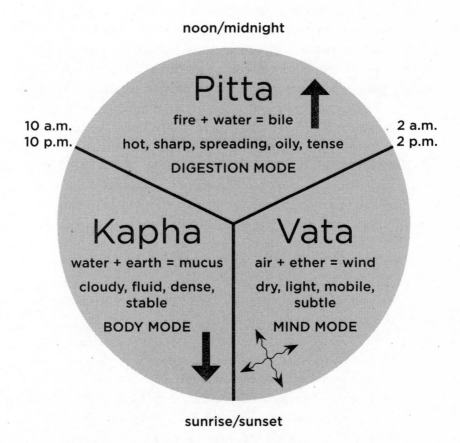

noon/midnight

Pitta

fire + water = bile

hot, sharp, spreading, oily, tense

DIGESTION MODE

10 a.m.
10 p.m.

2 a.m.
2 p.m.

Kapha

water + earth = mucus

cloudy, fluid, dense, stable

BODY MODE

Vata

air + ether = wind

dry, light, mobile, subtle

MIND MODE

sunrise/sunset

**The Three Energies
of the Human Body and Mind**

If you engage the second wind, you borrow against your tomorrow and incur a deficit. The deficit blows through your deep energy stores and then moves through your immune system. You need to optimize your biorhythms through listening to and honoring your body's subtle messages. Pay particular attention to the way your body communicates end-of-the-day fatigue. During kapha time, you should feel the impulse to let go and unwind. If you don't unwind, you'll be keyed up when you go to bed, and your sleep will be influenced by that energy. Like increases like. Instead, feel the downward pull of gravity. When you surrender to nature's body clock—which operates your organs and systems—better health, true energy, and immune integrity are within reach.

Research shows that when you go to bed late and don't get enough sleep, you train your body to produce cortisol around 8:00 p.m.[6] This stimulating hormone prevents you from winding down. You get pulled into a negative feedback loop that leads to massive endocrine disruption. Researchers of a sleep deprivation study found that "elevations of evening cortisol levels in chronic sleep loss are likely to promote the development of insulin resistance, a risk factor for obesity and diabetes."[7] Furthermore, sleep loss increases appetite that goes beyond what you need from the calories burned from staying up. It comes down to this: you need to wind down around 8:00 p.m. to experience deep sleep and deep fat burning, and to rebalance your endocrine system. When you don't do this, over time you mess with your endocrine system, which includes the stress hormone cortisol, your thyroid-stimulating hormone, and your growth hormone. Sleep researchers have identified a link between sleep deprivation and obesity:

> During the second half of the 20th century, the incidence of obesity has nearly doubled, and this trend is a mirror image of the decrease in self-reported sleep duration. The discovery of a profound alteration in the neuroendocrine control of appetite in conditions of sleep loss is consistent with the conclusions of several epidemiologic studies that revealed a negative association between self-reported sleep duration and body mass index. Taken together, the

current evidence suggests a possible role for chronic sleep loss in the current epidemic of obesity.[8]

If you're averaging six to seven hours of sleep, it's just flat-out dangerous. According to those CDC reports, short-changing your sleep over the long run leads to every disease, imbalance, and accident imaginable.[9] If you compound a sleep deficit night after night, you're in for costly, undesired, long-term problems.

Understanding Ojas and Immune Integrity

Ojas in Ayurveda is akin to the gel of our immune system. It's our subtle, refined energy. Ojas is an end product of excellent digestion and superior tissue formation. As such, the quality of our ojas reflects our consciousness and our choices. Ojas creates and protects the functional communication between all the cells and systems in our body. Integrity indicates coherence, shared identity, and unification, as well as stability, sturdiness, and durability. Cells perform many duties, including bringing in the groceries, taking out the trash, and talking to the neighbors, plus doing their specific job for their particular bodily system. The more your cells are working as an intelligent, unified whole, the more you experience excellent health and strong immunity.

Though repetitively violating any of the 10 Habits of Body Thrive can destroy ojas, the fastest way is to stay up late. If your habit is to burn the candle at both ends by emptying your inbox or watching your favorite drama or sports team, you will slowly destroy your ojas. Here are common lifestyle factors that disintegrate ojas:

- Being sleep deficient

- "Pushing through" fatigue instead of taking rest

- Overscheduling and overwhelm

- Using caffeine, sugar, or chocolate (including dessert) to get a first, second, or third wind

- Habitually worrying and stressing out

- Eating haphazardly instead of on a regular schedule

- Perpetuating unhealthy relationships

- Lacking self-confidence and indulging in negative self-talk

- Stagnation of bodily fluids from not enough daily movement

- Shallow breathing

Once you're aware of these factors, you can notice what you're perpetuating. Then you can inject a better habit sequence to put an end to the self-destruction.

Kaizen Your Bedtime to Build Ojas

The fastest way to build ojas is to dial in a peaceful, relaxing evening routine. If you ate an earlier, lighter dinner, you are sailing steady. If you ate a late, heavy dinner, you missed the boat.

With a simpler, early dinner, you have time to be active before bed. You'll settle your digestion, burn a few calories, and enjoy being in your body. My family likes to take a stroll, tend to the garden or house, or jump on the trampoline. If you feel stuck in your life or if you feel like time is not your own, you need to apply a kaizen approach to living in sync with your biorhythms.

What small habits will help you have the evenings you want? What will help you get the rest your body needs? Take a moment and review your typical evening routine—the one you default to when you don't break your own pattern. That one.

What is working for you? What do you *love* about it? Where is there room for improvement? Remember the most basic rule of habit evolution—take a small bite and chew well. Swallow. Repeat.

Here is a small bite for a revised evening routine: Right after you "close" the kitchen, rest on the couch for two minutes and relax into deeper, conscious breathing. Exhale the exhaustion of the day. Inhale refreshment. Drop into your body. If you'd rather lie down and close your eyes for a few minutes, do that. If you have fatigue, feel and drop into it instead of pulling away. Connect with your body. After two minutes, *visualize* the rest of your evening based on what your body wants and needs. This two-minute check-in practice restructures your evening with ease and flow. Maybe your body wants a walk, a bath, a hug, or just sleep. When you see what you want in your inner eye, you plant the seeds of future behavior.

If winding back your bedtime is difficult to do even in fifteen-minute increments, insert this body check-in habit before or after dinner. Pick a conscious choice-point, such as after the dinner dishes are done and you close your kitchen. You could use "kitchen closed" as your "preceding action" trigger. Then, insert your new habit.

Reverse-Engineer Deep Sleep

The early-to-bed habit doesn't start and end with bedtime. You should prepare yourself for better-quality rest, deep energy building, an easeful state of mind. By the end of the day, you have accumulated experiences, emotions, thoughts, and ideas. Give yourself some time to turn your attention inward, to process, and to wipe the slate clean before you rest. Combine this with an earlier, lighter dinner and not snacking between meals, and you'll experience the difference between waking up at 2:00 a.m. with new project ideas and concerns versus sleeping peacefully through the night to wake refreshed and energized. Basically, you want to go to bed with a clear head.

If your mind is a muscle that you can strengthen, your subconscious mind is like a malleable, swampy underworld that manipulates your thoughts, emotions, and habits. Use this to your advantage, or you may get sucked under by a monster. See in your mind's eye the path you want your subconscious to take the next day. Mentally rehearse when and how you'll rise, how you'll start your day, what you'll eat and drink, what you'll work on, when and how you will exercise and relax. This takes less than a minute and embeds better neural pathways. When you are falling asleep and when you first wake up, your mind is the most malleable—and so are your habit patterns. This tip aligns your life and neatens up the murky underworld in the easiest, most effortless way.

Enhance Your Sleep Habits and Habitat

If you're a light sleeper or you wake during the night, troubleshoot what is happening. If you are chronically stressed, you need to train your nervous system to wind down. If it's environmental, you can fix that.

Your bedroom is for sleeping. Is there too much light or sound? Are you disturbed by another person? If you want your sleep to be serene, your sleep habitat should be serene. Like increases like. Serenity increases serenity. Keep a clutter-free, stimulation-free room for sleep. Each morning, pick up your room so it feels like a sleep sanctuary. If you're having trouble sleeping, don't read in bed. Train yourself just to sleep in bed.

I use a black-out sleep mask because I'm ridiculously sensitive to light. If you're sensitive to sound, try squirting a little sesame oil on one side of a small cotton ball and inserting it into your ear, oily side first. This will bring your awareness inward while calming your sensitivity and deadening noise.

Furthermore, you want to sleep in alignment. Just as at the end of a yoga practice, when you lie in *Savasana*, or Corpse Pose, to absorb your practice, start your sleep sojourn by lying flat on your back, without a pillow, and simply absorb your day. Plant the mental pathways in your subconscious for tomorrow. Let the fatigue in your body and mind set in. Then, if you want to change positions, do so mindfully. Lying on your side or back is best. If you are a side sleeper, put a pillow between your knees to align your spine and hips. Stack your ankles. Use your pillow to keep your spine in line with your skull. If you lie on your back, slowly wean yourself off your pillow to avoid pushing your neck forward of your spine. Take a small-step approach to changing your sleep position so that you don't interrupt your sleep.

If you're prone to insomnia or interrupted sleep, employ an unwinding strategy. If I wake up in the middle of the night, I'll breathe deeply for a moment and then meditate while lying on my back. A simple strategy, like counting breaths and restarting at zero when your mind wanders, is an effective way to steer clear of feeding the fire of mental stimulation. If you chant a mantra, repeat it silently. Allow your awareness to take refuge in a calming practice, and you'll get some of the benefits of sleep. If insomnia is a repeated pattern, wean yourself from regular use of alcohol and caffeine. Switch to decaf and mineral water. Or make hot tea or golden milk, which is milk—nut or dairy—boiled with turmeric and spices such as ginger (to help you digest the milk) and nutmeg (to calm your nerves) before you sleep. Add honey as desired.

Tuning In with the "Ah" Breath

As a mom with a robust career, I'm not immune to the impulse to squeeze more out of every day. Yet at this point in the game, I rarely get pulled into the allure to get more done. The trick is to build in the triggers and habits so you don't stray far down the path of unintentional self-destruction.

When my daughter was a baby, we started this simple evening routine: I would prepare her for bed in the typical way of mothers and babies: bath, oil massage, and PJs. We would turn the lights low, read a few stories, snuggle in bed, and do "ah" breaths.

I first learned the power of the "ah" breath from the lovely meditation guru Sally Kempton. "Ah" is the most basic sound—the sound of the cosmos—emerging from the source and taking us back to our source.[10] It is the beginning of the three-part sound cycle of the cosmic *Aum* and the sound of the divine in any language. It's our vocalization of the big, wide, open of time and space. Try it and notice what happens to your mouth. Say the name of your favorite deity and see if you can find the long "aahhh" sound in their name. Here are a few: God, Buddha, Gaia, Allah, Yahweh, Inanna, Shiva, Shakti, Ram, Jehovah, Atman, Abba.

My daughter, Indy, and I lie in bed together, and I say, "Let's make the sound 'ah' as we breathe out. Now, let a big breath come in. See your belly rising? Now let's make a big sound from our big belly: 'Aaahhhh.'" And so it goes for ten slow, symphonic breaths.

My child and I have kept up this routine. She is normally a very active and social kid, and when she first gets into bed, she's still very keyed up. Our wind-down ritual includes "aahhhing." Because she has been trained with abhyasa almost every night of her life, she surrenders into the pattern. Without fail, after her third or fourth "aahhh," she yawns. Within a moment, she rubs her eyes, touches her face, or brings her special brown blankey around her neck and gets sucked into the beautiful abyss of peaceful sleep.

What does this have to do with you honoring your body's fatigue signals at the end of the day? Well, back in the early days of our nightly "ah" breath, I noticed that I, too, would drop into the deep drowsiness like a fly getting sucked up a vacuum.

With the "ah" breath, my exhale deepens. I breathe out the day's tensions and microstresses. If I'm tired, I get in touch with honest fatigue. When you're not resisting, fatigue is delish. I breathe my nerves into a relaxation response. Then I mentally rehearse a nourishing evening agenda. Some nights, I go to bed at the same time as my seven-year-old. Other nights, I relax, reflect, and renew with an enjoyable bedtime routine.

An Aromatic Love Affair

I love to use high-quality essential oils in my early-to-bed routine. The clean, potent plant aromas shift my mind by altering my emotions and enhancing my biochemistry. I rub coconut oil scented with lavender essential oil on my feet and the back of my neck when I want something light and airy. I use cedarwood when my mind is light and airy and I want to weigh it down for sleep. While I'm at it, I may rub clary sage over my ovaries, eucalyptus over my lungs, or, if I have sore butt muscles from challenging workouts, I'll use a wintergreen and peppermint blend. I dilute the essential oils with a base oil like coconut, sesame, or shea butter.

More important than the details is the concept—I have an aromatic love affair with my body and my senses before bed. The essential oils induce theta brain-wave states and deep relaxation, setting the tone for deep rebuilding and repair overnight.[11]

Essential oils work for me. This, or other conscious, body-loving, self-care routines, may work for you. The important practice is the investigation. What evening ritual gives you the deepest rest at this phase in your life? A bath? A walk? Restorative yoga? Meditation? Quiet contemplation? Journaling? Spiritual reading? Find a practice that helps you reflect and clear out the day to prepare for deep, restful sleep.

To follow through, see your future activities in your mind's eye. Visually walk yourself through a better bedtime routine. You are building a deep reservoir of energy in yourself. Your immune system will become more unified, strong, and stable. You'll be less prone to stress, accidents, relationship drama, and mindless decisions.

Be brutally honest with yourself because brutal honesty—or subtle transparency—is how consciousness works. If the universe of you is working great, you'll have insights into how to make it work even better. If it's not working, you will know why. Follow these habits until you know what works for how you want to feel.

Rules, Rigidity, and Flexibility

Do you need to go to bed by 10:00 p.m. every night? This depends on your health, your age, your goals, your desires. At certain phases in your life, that guideline may serve you. At other phases in your life, it may be impossible. Instead of setting yourself up for failure, see your daily habits in a larger context. And don't get hung up on making rules or promises that you can't keep.

I, like most, don't do well with rigid rules. If there is a rule, I break it just to challenge authority. But over time, I have learned it's wiser to conform to nature's rules, at least most of the time. Nature's rules are ever present and universal. You can't be separated from that out of which you arose. Yet, you can choose to make life better or worse for yourself. We are all free to choose exhaustion and overwhelm, again and again.

Take a moment and reflect: What is the middle road for you right now? What is a moderate bedtime? And how often can you break your moderate rule to live on the wild side and still be on track for your Body Thrive goals? It's unclear which wise person said, "Everything in moderation, including moderation," but they nailed it.

"Everything in moderation, including moderation." For my ojas-building, early-to-bed routine, moderation for me requires that I turn my switch off between 9:00 and 10:00 p.m. about six nights a week.

I've been dialing my bedtime back slowly over the years. Sometimes, particularly when I'm hitting a deadline or a big swell hits the shore, I dial bedtime back to 8:30 p.m. and rising to 4:30 a.m. Seriously. The more dynamic and compelling you want your life to become, the simpler your routines should be. When I'm leading a retreat or I'm at a big family gathering, I'll stay up later to connect for a few days. Then immediately after, I'll return to strict routines that meet my body's needs and long-term goals.

Early-to-Bed Identity Evolution

If you're a night owl, you may convince yourself that this is just how you are—you can't change, and you don't want to change. But have you seen the research? Night owls exercise less.[12] Night owls are notably more dangerous drivers.[13] Night owls drink and smoke more.[14] Other studies show that night owls are at greater risk of depression and experience worse sleep and more tiredness during the day—an experience researchers likened to a chronic form of jet lag.[15] Chronic jet lag? No, thank you.

Is your sleep pattern responsible for a muffin-top of fat storage and interrupted sleep? We need cortisol to handle emergencies, but not for reacting to email after 9:00 p.m. When cortisol is aligned to circadian rhythm, it peaks around 8:30 a.m., when you're getting fired up for action. By midnight, when you should be dropping into a deep sleep cycle, cortisol hits its low point. To balance cortisol in your circadian rhythm, you need to wind back bedtime and insert calming practices. Mess with your cortisol and risk acquiring a muffin top, because we now know that increased levels of cortisol lead to ugly fat deposits, particularly around the waist.[16]

The problem is, if you're like most night owls, you prefer to be a night owl rather than a bright-eyed, bushy-tailed morning person. Your persona, or *ahamkara*, is identified with your night-owlness, and those morning people are dorks who aren't in touch with the mystery of the night. I get it.

What keeps most night owls perpetuating their pattern is they self-identify with being night owls, consciously or subconsciously. They see it as a way to assert their independence, adultness, creativity, or rebellious nature. Saints, sages, and goody-two-shoes turn in early; artists and rebels revel into the wee hours.

A secret to shifting your habits is to update your identity in line with the next phase of what you want for yourself. Maybe you need to update your story of who goes to bed early. Successful people go to bed early. Healthy people go to bed early. See yourself as a successful, healthy person. Shift your identity to line up with your evolving goals for yourself. To do this, construct an updated identity for yourself.

To get clear on what needs to shift in your identity to turbocharge your better habits, fill out the Identity-Evolving Worksheet in the *Body Thrive Workbook* at bodythrive.com/free.

Once you're clear on your new identity, seek out comrades who also go to bed early. Let an early-bird friend or two know your intentions. Ask for encouragement and guidance. Strengthen who you are by cultivating a tribe of like-minded action-takers who will rub off on you.

TIPS FOR BUILDING OJAS BEFORE BED

- After dinner, talk a walk. Enjoy relaxed, connected family time. Play a game or do household chores that are slow-movement-oriented, like laundry or gardening. Schedule projects for another time. Be done by 8:00 p.m.

- Set a get-ready-for-bed alert on your phone.

- Keep lights dim after dinner.

- Eat dinner by candlelight once a week.

- Watch the sky change.

- If you have trouble sleeping soundly, stop using caffeine and alcohol. Switch to decaf, virgin spritzers, and herbal tea.

- Wind back your bedtime by fifteen-minute increments per week until you're getting eight hours of sleep a night.

- Set a curfew on some or all nights by turning off laptops, cell phones, televisions, tablets, and whatever device gets invented next.

- Meditate. Do breathing practice or restorative yoga.

- Take a bath or sit in a hot tub (preferably enzyme treated).

- Use calming essential oils like lavender and cedarwood; dilute them with a base oil of coconut, sesame, or sunflower.

- Journal about your day before bed.

- Sit or lie in Savasana for five minutes after you turn out the lights. Let your mind unwind and brain activity become quiet before you fall asleep. If this doesn't work, learn *yoga nidra* from YouTube or a local yoga teacher.

- After hosting visitors or traveling, get back to your routine.

HABIT 3

Start Your Day Right

WHAT TO DO

Take two minutes before you get out of bed to appreciate the coming day, see your life in a bigger context, and
mentally rehearse your better habits. Upon rising, drink
enough water to provoke complete elimination.

WHY YOU WANT TO DO IT

Train your perspective into the greater context of your
life, and you'll experience more connection, gratitude,
opportunities, and the freedom to design your life.
Make your life matter.

Before bed and upon arising, the neuroplasticity of
your mind is greatest. Set yourself up for the day you
want to have by mentally imprinting your choices and
your habits in line with who you want to become next
before the day gets ahead of you.

Waste in your channels will clog your whole day
and drag you down. Sufficient hydration activates your
bowels to empty, allowing you to enter your day fluid,
light, and clear. You'll experience more energy, clarity,
and flexibility.

HOW TO START

When you first awaken, expand your perspective and rehearse your day ahead. Start with drinking a cup of water, between room temperature and hot, as soon as you rise. Over time, increase this to a quart, or enough to stimulate a bowel movement.

Think of yourself as polar. The north pole is your crown—the top of your head. The south pole is your root—at the base of your spine. We're organized both physically and subtly around this north-south gravitational axis. The main energy channel of the subtle body is the *sushumna nadi,* the channel that connects consciousness through the subtle nervous system on a gravitational north-south axis. When the physical channel isn't eliminating well, expect problems in the subtle channel, which includes your inner state—your mind, thoughts, and emotions—and influences your relationships.

The main channel of the *physical* body is what we're focusing on here—the *maha vaha srota,* or the channel that connects the mouth to the anus. *Maha* means "great." *Vaha* is "to carry or move." *Srota* means "channel." This channel is the *raja,* or king, of the physical channels. Your duty as a human being is to flush your great channel before you bring any new experiences into your day or indigestibles to your gut, other than water.

Flush Your Inner Toilet

Each day you have a chance for a fresh start. A fresh start means deep-tissue hydration and a big poop. Around eighteen inches of eliminated fecal matter dumped within an hour of rising, without caffeine for provocation, is the gold standard. Deep hydration is prerequisite for healthy elimination, which is a requisite for your body to thrive. Once you're up and at 'em, sip or guzzle about a quart of water, between room temperature and tea-water hot. The purpose of this water is to flush your inner toilet.

I was constipated until I dialed in this habit of deep hydration and clockwork elimination. For me, if a quart of hot water doesn't pull the trigger, I drink another pint to flush my inner toilet. Seriously. This took some getting used to, but I went from a constipated chica to an authoritative pooping champion.

You want to empty the contents of both the descending colon and your transverse colon (the section that goes across your abdomen). A squatting stool sets your colon in alignment to release. Complete elimination releases *apana vayu*, the downward-flowing energy, and gives rise to *prana*, the upward-flowing energy. Upon releasing apana vayu, you will feel a flush of prana, or life force, as a scintillation in your colon.

At this point, if you pause, you can feel the connection between the physical and subtle body channels. You will feel like a champ—the rock star that you are—full of space, full of potential; the day will spread out before you.

You may start to see at this point how krama, including your bowel habits, either sets you up for a bigger, more on-purpose life or shoots you in the foot. Carry poop into your day, and your day will be soiled from the inside out.

One of the members in my Living Ayurveda Course had had chronic constipation since childhood. For as far back as she could remember, Kumari hadn't pooped like a champ. The pot was her battlefield. Food seemed to get stuck in her system, and only rabbit pellets emerged from the other end. Bloated and uncomfortable, she wanted help.

After Kumari heard me teach the how-to-flush-your-inner-toilet makeover a handful of times, she started upping her water intake in the morning and implementing the troubleshooting suggestions below. Her progress was slow, but it was progress.

When you uproot a deep imbalance, it's like uprooting a tree. Put down your chainsaw and take time to dig at the roots to bring down the tree of imbalance. After six months, Kumari reports that she now poops like a pro. Like clockwork. She joined my Pooping Champions Who Used to Be Constipated Club.

To motivate you to master this habit, here are six benefits of healthy, complete elimination:

- Your colon absorbs nutrients better.

- Your metabolism is stronger, and it's easier to balance your body weight.

- Your cells hydrate faster, which helps in production of blood and muscle cells.

- You have a working exit for ama.

- Your skin may glow because you have less waste in circulation.

- Your lymphatic circulation improves, which improves your immune function.

Troubleshoot Your Poop

If you're fired up to poop but your innards are stuck or unpredictable and loose, troubleshoot it. If you're already eating an earlier, lighter dinner and drinking your morning water, you may need more specific suggestions. Evaluate your habits for anything missing in your daily routine. Do you:

- Eat a clean, whole-foods diet with lots of nonstarchy vegetables and leafy greens?

- Drink water almost exclusively? (Habitual caffeine and alcohol intake will dehydrate your bowels.)

- Eat a more liquid diet with green smoothies, soups, and stews to keep your feces hydrated?

- Space your meals with only water in between two or three meals a day?

- Have fermented foods in your regular diet?

If you've had bowel issues for decades, the imbalance can be slow to uproot. An Ayurvedic teacher once told me, for every year you've had an imbalance, it can take a month to uproot. To extrapolate, if you've had elimination irregularity for a decade, it may take close to a year to shift your bowels into regularity. Cleansing or rejuvenating your colon as needed through detox, *panchakarma* (Ayurvedic cleansing), enemas, colonics, herbal formulas, diet appropriate for your constitution and type of digestion, and yoga can alleviate the most stubborn cases of bowel issues. Here are some basic suggestions for constipation:

- Use a squatting stool, like a Squatty Potty. Unkink your colon when you poop.

- Eat a more liquid diet with green juices, smoothies, soups, and stews. Avoid crackers, breads, and starchy foods—even starchy vegetables, which require a lot of water to eliminate.

- If you haven't gone by the time you're hungry, make a fresh juice or smoothie with beets, cucumbers, apples, celery, and parsley.

- Try stewed apples for dessert or for breakfast.

- Eat roasted, stewed, or pickled beets regularly.

- Soak chia seeds in a Mason jar in your fridge and add a scoop to your morning cereal or smoothie.

- Switch to decaf, or wean entirely from caffeine, which weakens natural peristalsis over time.

- Try a magnesium supplement (like Natural Calm) before bed.

- Take Downward-Flow (available from Yogahealer.com) for occasional constipation.

- Take Colon-Repair (available from Yogahealer.com) for chronic constipation.

- Take the Ayurvedic herb *triphala* by itself or mixed with castor oil; it's very effective for stubborn constipation.

Here are some basic suggestions for loose stools:

- Add the juice from half a lime to your morning water.

- Mix bilva, slippery elm, licorice root, and triphala. Take before bed. Or try the herbal blend called Elim 2 (available from LifeSpa.com).

- Mix ¼ cup of plain yogurt with the same amount of water and ⅛ teaspoon of nutmeg. Add a pinch of salt or sweetener as desired. Take after meals. Or, sprinkle nutmeg on meals.

- Eat underripe bananas.

Notice what works, and stick to it as you add modalities to optimize your absorption and elimination.

Breaking the Pearl Necklace

When I was learning *pranayama* while in the Iyengar yoga teacher training for two years, our teacher stressed the necessity of daily practice. Repetition, daily, over time, is like stringing pearls for a necklace. Skip a day and the chain is broken, and you need to start building momentum again.

Travel, stress, and transitions of any sort aggravate constipation. Knowing this, be diligent about forming world-class bowel habits so you don't drop the ball. William James's wisdom from his 1890 book, *Habit*, applies today:

Never suffer an exception to occur till the new habit is securely rooted in your life. Each lapse is like the letting fall of a ball of string which one is carefully winding up; a single slip undoes more than a great many turns will wind again. Continuity of training is the great means of making the nervous system act infallibly right.[1]

In the first hours of the day—the time before the dawn—there is a unique opportunity. The yogis named this precious grace-filled period *brahmamuhurta*. In the twenty-four-hour cycle, this is the time that is most peaceful, most easeful, and has the easiest access to the sacred. It's the gorgeous, quiet early hours. If you awake and attune, your neural pathways are the most malleable. Historically, spiritually oriented humans have heeded a basic desire to connect with our being-ness, our self beyond time and space, during this time.

The ancient Ayurvedic text, *Ashtanga Hridayam*, states: "The healthy person should get up during brahmamuhurta, to protect his life."[2] This statement comes early in the text for priority and doesn't mince words: waking early protects your life.

The earliest hours of your day offer a unique opportunity to align your life by aligning your mindset. Sleep through the early dawn, and your mind and body will be more dense—your spirit less plugged into your form. The fifteenth-century Indian mystic Kabir poetically expounds:

O friend, awake, and sleep no more!
The night is over and gone, would you lose your day also?
Others who have wakened, have received jewels[3]

Kabir lays to rest the argument that many creative night owls make. He divides us into winners and losers: those who wake early and find, compared to those who sleep in and lose. This black-or-white approach to Start the Day Right happens with habit automation.

Brahmamuhurta is a humble, wise time. Around the world, masses of people start the day in prayer. A global tribe of meditators bows their heads before embarking into practice. They bow to release head to heart, to release separateness into unity. Kabir points to waking, opening your eyes, and meditating on your master.

The key to the Start Your Day Right habit is to attune your attention with a specific practice or action, to intentionally meld your body-mind-spirit into cosmocentric consciousness. This is the master, the higher will, the universal intelligence we have the most access to at a specific time of day: the dawn. Do this, and you'll not only experience more of the flow state in your day, you'll also live a life aligned to your potential. I've found particular practices helpful for various stages of my life. Over the years, I've engaged in a variety of practices to attune myself to brahmamuhurta. I've used meditation, pranayama, prayer, chanting, writing, yoga, and inquiry practice. I don't get attached to the practice itself, but rather to the commitment to a daily practice that widens my perspective, increases connectivity, or accesses higher planes of insight.

Engage the Sacred

To see the importance of Start Your Day Right, meet Jasmine, a mom with teenagers. She joined the Body Thrive coaching program because she felt like her life was slipping by without her steering from the helm. Her family role was shifting as her children were close to flying the coop. Over the years, she had lost connection with her deeper desires, with what she wanted in her life. She felt a little depressed, a little overweight, and was just keeping up with the day-to-day.

When I asked Jasmine about her bedtime and morning routines, she told me the typical modern story of staying up late catching up on email, browsing the web, or watching the big-screen TV with her family. She would "fiddle around the house" and tidy up until past 11:00 p.m. She was disturbed from deep sleep by her alarm at 6:00 a.m. Her days began in a sequence of catch-up to get the family and herself out the door. She was underslept. She needed to go to bed earlier if she was ever going to tap into the power of brahmamuhurta.

I asked Jasmine to start winding back her bedtime. She was serious about change, so I recommended a 9:30 p.m. lights out and a 5:00 to 5:30 a.m. wake-up. She could have taken her time adjusting her rhythms, but she was ready for abrupt change. We structured a very simple routine for her to do upon arising, including hydrating, eliminating, and a mind-body movement practice. At first, her practice consisted of five Sun Salutations and five minutes of prayer, which she loved doing as a child.

After two weeks of strictly sticking to her new routine, Jasmine craved her morning ritual. She wanted more of what she named "divine time" to herself. As she committed to her divine time, she experienced an inner peace that became an accessible backdrop to her whole day. She had an inner knowing that this simple practice would slowly reveal the next phase of her life, aligned. She started to feel light, alert, and uplifted.

Then family came to visit. She stayed up late, and she missed her morning ritual for several days. The depression and heavy feeling came back in full force. She was surprised at the depth of desire to return to her new routine.

Often this is the case. When you've aligned for even a short period of time and then regress, you more clearly experience the impact of misaligned choices. It may feel like your more enlightened self is telling you, "I told you so!"

With the habit of greeting brahmamuhurta well rested and alert, you engage the sacred. What you do then is secondary to how you approach this time of day. During this brief time in the twenty-four-hour cycle, you are the most pliant, free, and expansive, most available to dive into spirit. Imprint your consciousness with a big perspective of your life, and zoom out on what matters most. Take time to align—from the big picture to your specific daily actions—as you zoom in on what should happen on a particular day. And remember, when you want to get more sleep, go to bed earlier. Sleeping in only sets you up for going to bed later the next night.

Early Mornings and Your Mood

When I work with depressed clients, my first question is "What time do you go to bed and wake up?" With rare exceptions, the person is a night owl or has an irregular sleep schedule. Typically, mornings begin with coffee and mental, but not physical, activity such as reading the news or tackling email. This is not good.

There is a basic Ayurvedic practice for depression based on brahmamuhurta: take a walk facing the rising sun. It's easy to see why that works. If you walk to meet the rising sun, you witness the miracle, the dawning of a new day. The metaphor subtly awakens the possibility of your life. By igniting your inner light, you burn off the fog of depression.

Plus, you're exercising, which is proven to alleviate depression and improve brain function and brain-cell growth.[4] All this is happening first thing—infusing your emotional day with the natural, life-positive default mode that comes from living in alignment. Do this daily and your negative emotions will cease to get the better of you.

When I work with anxiety-ridden clients, I also press the issue of bedtime and waking time. Time and again, their sleep/wake schedule doesn't follow Ayurveda's recommended daily rhythm. These people haven't made time to meditate or breathe before their day begins. As they move their bedtime and waking time backward on the clock, space and time are freed up. They learn to integrate a peaceful morning ritual that anchors serenity into their brain chemistry. They rewire their perspective to get grounded in their body, in time, and in space. Anxiety dissipates. Calm settles in like clockwork.

Commit to being awake and well rested for the daily miracle of your life—when darkness transitions into light. Use whatever practice, ritual, or habit flips your switch. Try gratitude practice, prayer, meditation, mantra—whatever pulls your trigger. Go to where the juice is for you. Plus, like most good habits, it's free and prerequisite for living a life aligned.

Wake Up to Your Potential

After many months, Jasmine checked in with me. She had started a small club with her girlfriends who had been in the same boat of feeling off track and unfulfilled. They created a commitment club for going to bed early, waking up early, and doing a morning practice, each in their own homes. Once a week, they would meet for lunch and discuss how they were designing the next phase of their lives, one day at a time. They would deeply listen to each other and offer encouragement, accountability, and guidance.

Jasmine informed me she'd enrolled in a professional training program that lit her up. She was reshaping her career. Her eyes sparkled as her passion revealed itself to her. She regretted the many years she'd drifted through her life. She was mystified at how one habit was able to keep her on track with who she felt destined to become. Let's look at why this basic shift in daily rhythms and practices upgraded Jasmine's life.

When you live exclusively in what the yogis call the "waking state," or gross reality, you miss the subtle, behind-the-scenes, always-already-arising deep mystery of life. You get locked in the mundane. You may even take the basics for granted: water, food, shelter, clean air, electricity, cars, paved roads, green smoothies, your body, mind, emotions, relationships—the list goes on.

As the poet Rumi wrote, "Darkness is your candle. / Your boundaries are your quest."[5] Every divine tradition points to your immortal nature—your self beyond time and space. When you're awake for brahmamuhurta, you are between worlds. The veils between subtle and gross lift. The sense of the whole, of fullness, fulfillment, and perfection, are within reach.

Fill Your Own Cup First

The word for the experience of deep fulfillment in yoga is *purnima* or *purna*, which describes the feeling of the fullness of the full moon. The yogis' teaching of purna is that your true nature is intrinsically deeply satisfied, deeply contented. Purna encompasses your limitations, your contractions, and even your endless striving to become more. Your being nature is already perfect and complete. Experiencing this optional reality of being-ness sets your nervous system into a baseline of relaxed expansion for the day. You fill you own inner cup first and are ready for action from a place of inner wholeness.

Although the experience of purna is always already here, right now, for many of us it is inaccessible. This means that your day takes off in a trajectory of endless to-dos, and your nerves are patterned into a stress response. Like anything that is out of reach, you simply need a plan of small steps to bring it within reach. The questions become: How do you start the day right? How do you jump off the stress-mobile and walk into the zone?

Almost all of us wake up in the "me"-centric perspective George Harrison so eloquently voiced in the Beatles song "I Me Mine." The sacred morning practice to align with the divine trains your perspective to experience the fullness of the cosmos, of deep time, of deep space. Train your perspective into gratitude for your body, for the planet, for the air you breathe at the start of each day. Train your perspective to attune to the naturally expansive energy dominant in the time before the sun has risen. Ether element, a component of the pre-sunrise *vata* energy, dominates this phase of the twenty-four-hour cycle. When you rise before the sun, your awareness will naturally attune and expand. You'll feel time open up. You won't be as busy, rushed, or unorganized that day. Your early mornings beget deeper fulfillment and an easeful flow in your daily life. This is why Kabir wrote, "He who awakes, he finds." And conversely, "One who is asleep, he loses."

To step into a bigger perspective, a bigger dharma, a bigger life—to "be all you can be"—engage with a practice before or around 6:00 a.m. Align your day with a perspective that places your current reality in the inconceivable context of the absolute perfection of the imperfect now. Receive who you are becoming.

To download Audio Meditation: Return to Zero, an audio of a guided meditation to start your day in a bigger perspective, visit body thrive.com/free.

TIPS TO START THE DAY RIGHT

- Go to bed earlier so you can wake up earlier. Don't mess with your ability to be an awake, connected, healthy human being.

- Pray, give gratitude, or do a meditation practice that expands your perspective beyond the "I-me-my" mental tendency.

- Envision the day ahead. Visualize specific actions in line with whom you wish to become.

- Wake up and hydrate with fresh water—preferably room temperature to almost tea-water hot—if you tend toward constipation.

- Train your bowels to eliminate in the early morning. Give yourself time to poop before the day gets away from you. Use a squat stool.

- Don't give up on the dream of regular morning elimination. The Yoga Health Coaches hear of such miracles happening to the least likely people every day.

HABIT 4

Bestir Your Breath-Body

WHAT TO DO

After your morning poop session, take twenty minutes
to move and groove to open up your body. Infuse your
cells with oxygen and invigorate your body into resil-
iency and power with breath-coordinated exercise before
you head out into your workday.

WHY YOU WANT TO DO IT

After sleeping all night, your body is stiff, blood oxygen
levels are low, blood flow is stagnant, and every cell is
in need of a shakedown and a sprucing up. Happy cells
have dynamic and integrated pulsation. Upon arising,
your vibration is stagnant and dull. Shake that off and
build a strong vibrational field for the day ahead. Air
out your breath channels and ignite your physical body
through coordinating your breath into movement. You'll
feel light, grounded, energized, open, and in your body
instead of in your head. Also, as you age, you want to
build a repertoire of skills that strengthen and nurture
your muscular-skeletal structure.

HOW TO START

Before breakfast, move and breathe deeply for at least
five minutes. Start with any kind of movement you
enjoy: walk; dance; stretch; stair-step; do jumping jacks,
mobility exercises, or burpees; swing a kettlebell; salute
the sun. Mix it up. Move from your breath, inhaling
and exhaling deeply and fully through your nose. If you
already have a movement-breath morning discipline,
expand your skills to enhance how you age with the
practices outlined below.

To be alive is to move. Life vibrates. Life pulsates. Disease stagnates.
Stagnation in your breath and blood breed the diseases of stagnation, which are omnipresent in Western culture. Any substance in
your body that is in excess or not moving becomes a breeding ground
of toxicity or a dead zone that sucks energy instead of generating
energy. According to Eastern medicine, stagnation is a root cause of
chronic and degenerative diseases, from diabetes to cancer to obesity.
Stagnation happens when prana, or energy in the body, isn't flow-
ing. Stagnation is common with eating too much or too frequently
and not moving enough. There is a new category of diseases in Western medicine now, termed "sedentary" diseases. These are diseases of
stagnation. Waking up to coffee and a computer is the recipe for stagnation and inflammation.

You want to wake up, release your waste (Habit 3), then uplevel your
vibration and bust any stagnation in your blood, in your joints, and even
in your emotional body. Ayurveda has terms that diagnose and shift
energies. When you wake up, you're *tamasic*, or stagnant. You use *rajas*,
or heat-generating action, and prana, or life-giving breath, to break up
the duller vibration and infuse the blood with *sattva*, or a higher vibratory field. You want to align your body and mind to meet the day at the
edge of your potential, instead of lugging around an oxygen-deprived
body and mind.

When you add Habit 4 to Habit 3, you wake up, hydrate, poop, and move daily, with no exceptions. Once you have this breath-body habit of arranging five to twenty minutes of movement or deep breathing into your pre-breakfast routine, your body will never want to give it up. You'll be hungry for a healthy breakfast, clear minded, inspired, relaxed, energized, and much more comfortable in your body.

The breath-body habit may be your exercise workout or a body-centric spiritual practice. A few components are required:

1. Do it every day after hydrating, and before eating or caffeinating.

2. Work up to a daily, twenty-minute session.

3. Connect movement to breath.

Even if you normally work out a few times a week after work, add this twenty-minute home routine. This habit insists you move *every* morning—before you eat, before you check email, before your day gets away from you—regardless of later-in-the-day athletic activities, trips, holidays, family reunions, or temporal chaos in your life. Some days you'll want to do a longer workout, some days shorter. Regardless, every morning you need to alchemize tamas into sattva. Early morning breath-centered movement is nonnegotiable for body thrive.

By gorging on oxygen, you enable your brain to make better decisions. Daily choices—what to feed yourself, who to spend time with, what to do with your time—have drastic, compounding consequences on your life and your health. The breath, or prana, carries more than oxygen. Prana also carries consciousness, which is infused with intelligence. The authors of a 2013 study on exercise and executive functioning reported, "Short bouts of exercise increase blood flow to the area of the brain responsible for executive brain functions, like making decisions or planning ahead and keeping one's cool."[1] By being aware of breathing and filling up with the breath, you deliver this intelligence into your lungs, and from there into your blood. Your heart pumps the intelligence-infused blood throughout your body, and your cells experience more energy, more connection, and awakened intuition. Think of it this way: prana makes your cells smarter, healthier, and superfunctional. From extensive research, you know you want your brain cells on exercise. When you're evolving your habits, you need to make better decisions. To make better decisions, you need your brain and the rest of your body infused with oxygen, consciousness, and energy for action.

Partnering with your breath is the name of the game. Yoga has a long-standing obsession with breath awareness and breath expansion in a practice called *pranayama*. Discussed in more detail in Habit 7, Sit in Silence, pranayama teaches the breathing practices that both stand alone and are part of yoga. You'll want to get the benefits of deep, conscious breathing in order to optimize your morning exercise. The Kripalu Center for Yoga and Health website explains:

> The aim of both yoga in general, and pranayama in particular, is to help us participate in the nearly unlimited intelligence of the life force so that we can share in its capacities. Instead of fighting nature, we gradually become able to partner with it. When the ancient seers began their study of the potential of being human thousands of years ago, they soon saw that working with the breath could yield impressive results toward greater aliveness, self-expression, and power. The breath is one of the easiest doorways into the capabilities of the human nervous system because it touches every aspect of our being: physical, physiological, psycho-emotional, and spiritual.[2]

This means you should become master of your breath as you age. You should become more adept with breath to unlock your personal wellness and growth path. You want to train your habits to tap into the power of a before-breakfast breath-body practice. Make every day awesome, and become more skillful as you age. Let's look at how to start.

At yoga class, you learn how to breathe deeply and coordinate movement with breath. You may have heard the effective instruction, "Let your breath initiate movement." Experiment with this, no matter what exercise you choose in the morning; the practice trains you to connect with life force first. *Let thy will be my will* is the experience of when you train your body to move from your breath. Allow your breath to initiate your action.

Years ago, I was at a weekend skate-skiers' party in Yellowstone with a group of friends. One of the dads, named Sage, whizzed around the hilly course where the US Cross Country Ski Team practices. None of us could keep up with him. For those who haven't skate skied, it's a full-body cardio extravaganza. As we were sitting around the fire later, I asked Sage to demonstrate how he breathed while skating.

Always animated, Sage widened his cheeks and flared his nostrils and nasal cavity. His face looked untamed, mammalian. He breathed through both nose and mouth simultaneously, directing oxygen deep into his torso. He said, "I try to get more oxygen any way I can. This is what works." Since then, I've been practicing Sage's pranayama technique when I ride my bike up mountains or propel my distance paddleboard through the wind.

Infuse Your Blood with Prana

Your breath offers a pathway into your organs for energy, consciousness, and cosmic intelligence. In your breath-body habit, you don't want to just move your limbs around, though that is a halfway decent starting place. You want to move your limbs from your "breath body" or "pranic body." Deep, coordinated breathing causes your blood, viscera, and limbs to become integrated, which grants access to your pranic body. Pulsing, rhythmic movement, like Sun Salutations or deep-breathing practices unlock deeper levels of body integrity or integration. The yogic subtle-body anatomy system—including the *chakras* (energy vortexes) and *nadis* (energy channels)—becomes more apparent, accessible, and tangible from the regular habits of early-morning breath-body practices. When you move your body from your breath, you enter a flow state that shallow breathing can't access. Our cells crave breath-centered movement because it partners mind and body while clearing stagnation and combusting disease and inflammation.

Finished before breakfast, this simple habit takes about twenty minutes, clears stagnation from the body, and infuses your body with energy, your mind with clarity, and your emotions with ease for an uplifted day.

Design Your Breath-Body Practice

You want to set yourself up for long-term success. If you don't currently move before you get on with your day or leave the house in the morning, start with five minutes of movement coordinated with deep breathing. Anything from a brisk, deep-breathing walk to yoga Sun Salutations will do the trick. The key is to train your body to get up and breathe deeply, moving from the breath.

Use behavior psychologist B. J. Fogg's statement: *"Right after I _____, I will _____."* Here is my example from this morning: "Right after I poop, I will do fifteen Sun Salutations and then swing a kettlebell for ten minutes."

Many people fail by inventing obstacles to get in the way of the breath-body movement habit. They forget about kaizen and bite off more than they can chew. This just may be your keystone habit, so don't make your regiment too hard or too long. You'll experience more energy throughout the day, *even* if your breath-body practice is five minutes long. Your statement may be: "Right after I poop, I will do two Sun Salutations and then jump rope for three minutes."

You'll make better choices throughout your day, as your body will be more intelligent without stagnation. You'll crave more movement and be more likely to take short, reenergizing walks or engage in quick bursts of intense movement, which we know optimize executive function.

Which exercise or breath-work practice you choose is less important than having this habit for the rest of your days. There are two inverse strategies for making a big shift:

1. Trust your interest—it's intelligent and evolving.

2. Do the opposite.

Either way can work. If you are psyched and know what you want to commit to, start there. Or do the opposite, as made famous by the *Seinfeld* episode in 1994 by that name:

> **George**   It became very clear to me sitting out there today, that every decision I've ever made, in my entire life, has been wrong. My life is the opposite of everything I want it to be. Every instinct I have, in every aspect of life, be it something to wear, something to eat . . . it's all been wrong.

> **Jerry**   If every instinct you have is wrong, then the opposite would have to be right.[3]

Ayurveda taps into the universal law of polarity, which states that opposites reduce each other. When you're out of thrive—for instance if you aren't moving enough—the opposite will help: move more! As you come into deeper thrive, your instincts will guide you deeper into thrive. Ayurveda states that with the universal law of the increase, "like increases like." In the following section, look at how to get the kind of physique, stamina, and flexibility you want by using the opposites of your tendencies and leveraging the good movements that you've already dialed in.

Hardening, Softening, and Cardio Workouts

Our bodies thrive on diversity of movement. So far we've learned that how we breathe matters and that we need to increase our breath capacity as we move.

I was taught by many a yoga "guru" to practice yoga for an hour every morning. For many years, I did twenty to seventy minutes of yoga *asanas* (postures) almost every morning. I was prejudiced against cross-training and weight training. My morning practice remained faithful to yoga.

Yet eventually I found my attention drifting off the mat. Desiring a change of pace, I strayed from the path, replacing asanas with cardio cross-training and functional movement, yoga blocks with kettlebells, and yoga straps with Indian clubs. Places where energy and cellulite had been stagnant started releasing. Cellulite melted. My body changed. When open places got tight, I needed my yoga practice again to open up my body, coordinate my limbs into unity consciousness, and center my soul. I fell back in love with my yoga because I needed it to balance the intensity from cross-training. I missed coordinated consciousness. At that point, I intuitively developed a sweet repertoire of breath-body practices and workouts to design the body, mind, emotions, and day I want to experience.

We can divide exercise into three categories: hardening, softening, and cardio. Integrative physician Eric Grasser, a favorite guest speaker in my Living Ayurveda course, designated three categories of exercise: ones that strengthen, soften, and sustain. He recommends "a triple combination of resistance training balanced with a slow, supportive, breath-controlled modality such as yoga movement, tai chi, dance, or something similar, rounded off with endurance movement."[4]

Hardening, or strength-building, workouts make your body strong and hard through contracting your muscles under pressure. Softening practices make your body flexible, open, soft, and pliant through stretching your muscles. Cardio, or sustaining practices, focus on pumping blood and moving your booty. Most of us have tendencies to prefer certain types of workouts. Which do you prefer?

Martial arts, Pilates, and yoga do the best job at mixing all three categories. However, done exclusively, they will also lead to mental stagnation as you fall into patterned learning. They are in the "softening" category because, when compared to other workouts, they have the most attention to breath, which softens and opens the body.

If you only follow your preference, you probably won't strategically mix hardening, softening, and cardio throughout the week. You risk less energy, more injury, faster aging, and less balance in your life.

Here is a brief list of different workouts—or "work-ins"—to help you evaluate your exercise tendencies. Of course, most activities will cross categories, but you want to look at the overall benefits and side benefits of your workouts. Notice which ones fall into the category you frequent versus frequently avoid:

Hardening Workouts

Weightlifting, kettlebells, Indian clubs, and weight training

CrossFit

Plyometrics or tactical bodyweight training (Tabata)

Push-ups, sit-ups, burpees, and other repetitive exercises

Running and repetitive-movement sports

Softening Workouts

Breath work, including pranayama

Mobility exercises

Martial arts, tai chi, or qigong

Yoga

Pilates, barre

Stretching

Dance

Cardio Workouts

Running

CrossFit

Dance

Boxing

Plyometrics

Metabolic conditioning

Basketball, soccer, tennis, Ultimate Frisbee, etc.

Surfing, paddleboarding, biking

Jumping rope, jumping jacks, push-ups, sit-ups, burpees, and other dynamic exercises

Intense movement, including all sports that get your heart rate up and your breath pumping

The idea is to cross-train in all three categories. All work and no play makes Jack a dull boy. It also gives Jack a dull body. Hardness leads to its own stagnation, blocking flexibility in body and mind, and limiting circulation, which results in injury.

All flow and no intense work makes Jack a doughboy. It makes Jack too soft and mellow. Softening practices unchecked can lack the deep cardio and buildup of muscular power, which gives embodied stature. Done incorrectly, softening exercise leads to hyper-flexibility and lack of mental direction.

All cardio is okay for Jack, but not great. He won't build deeper strength, and he'll lose muscle tone as he ages. He risks injury. Cardio practices strain muscles and wear out joints, tendons, and ligaments when not balanced by softening practices that lengthen the muscles, release lactic acid, and counterbalance repetitive motion.

Many dis-eases—including digestive issues, heart attacks, heart problems, athletic injury like muscle and tendon pulls, and even infertility, PMS, and menopause imbalances—are affected by not knowing how to mix these practices to fit your current body needs at this particular phase in your life. Take a moment and reflect on the following questions:

- What do you gravitate toward? Hardening, softening, or cardio workouts?

- What does your body need more of?

- How can you make that a habit this week?

- Print the Workout Chart from the *Body Thrive Workbook* at bodythrive.com/free. Fill in which days you'll do hardening, softening, and cardio. Strategically mix your workouts for a vibrant, strong, open body.

Challenging, Moderate, Easy Intensity

Another essential tool to balance your practice is to vary the intensity. Schedule hard, moderate, and easy workouts in your calendar, with no more than two to three challenging workouts a week. We all need hardening, softening, and cardio workouts. We all need challenging, moderate, and easy workouts in our schedule. Identify your gaps and the opposites of your tendencies. Add these to your Workout Chart.

Refer back to the section "Architect Your Choices" on page 27 to kick-start your new habits. For example, if you have a hard, cardio, weight workout scheduled tomorrow morning, set out your shoes, your weights, and whatever else you need for the workout you will be doing. This also reflects B. J. Fogg's model: get specific, make it easy, and trigger the behavior. You want to carve a path for your feet to follow each day. Soon the path becomes your daybreak superhighway.

Work Out Your Constitution

In Ayurveda, we could break this down further and design workouts to suit our constitution, or *dosha*: *vata*, *pitta*, or *kapha*. At this point, take a moment to identify your constitution with the Ayurvedic Constitution Quiz: bodythrive.com/quiz. When you know your Ayurvedic constitution, you can refine your breath-body practices to meet your unique needs.

We're all built with the same building blocks, but in different proportions. From the Ayurvedic perspective, everyone has all five elements (ether, air, fire, water, and earth) and all three energetic forces that make up our unique constitutions (pitta, vata, kapha), but in different proportions.

Vatas are our celestial featherweights. Delicate and sensitive, they require subtler practices than their bigger-boned counterparts. Trying to fit in, Vatas often risk injury and depletion to hang with the mid- and heavyweights. Vatas proportionally need more softening, restorative practices, and more easy-to-moderate workouts than the other body types.

If your constitution is predominately vata—which has more catabolic (breaking-down) energy—design your breath-body practices to increase metabolic (transformative) and anabolic (building) energies. That way you won't wear yourself out or tear yourself up. To translate that into hardening, softening, and cardio, you'll focus more on softening, which will help you build tissue, and cardio, which will stimulate metabolism.

In contrast, Kaphas, our earthly heavyweights, are built to endure rough conditions and tolerate intensity. Although tough to get moving, once in motion, Kaphas stay in motion. Kaphas can be very complacent about their bigger bodies, easily slipping into couch-potato land. These types need cardio and hardening practices, with more moderate-to-challenging workouts on the weekly schedule. Kaphas often need an accountability partner to stimulate their complacency into action.

Pittas, our fiery middleweights, will want to act like a Kapha due to their intense ambition, but can get injured or burned out in the process. Pittas need equal time with hardening, softening, and cardio. When out of balance due to burnout, Pittas can often use more softening, easy, restorative workouts. However, their tendency is to use their mental ambition to deplete their bodies.

Play around with your exercise workouts. Balance strengthening your body with opening your body. Experiment and determine what fitness schedule works best for you in this cycle of your life. Be curious. Notice the effects. Let your body uncover the truth of what is working and what you need next.

If you always do yoga, try CrossFit or swing a kettlebell. If you run, try dancing. If you dance, run. If you lift weights, stretch. If you stretch, lift. If you work out indoors, go outside. Challenge yourself. Build a repertoire. As Joseph Campbell famously reminds us from the grave: *"Follow your bliss."* What do you want to add to upgrade how fit you are?

If you need training on what you want to add, find a live teacher, a training video on YouTube, or a course on the web. Check the Hard, Moderate & Easy Workouts tip sheet in the *Body Thrive Workbook*. Before bed, set out what you need for your morning practice. Before sleep, visualize getting yourself to your morning workout and digging in.

Again, it's just before the dawn. You wake up. You want to roll over. You are at a choice point—the very first choice of your day. Will you hydrate, take out the trash, and blow out the stagnation to have a truly vibrant day? Take small steps. Set yourself up for the long game in a fit, alert body and mind. Become fascinated with what your body craves as it wakes up to new levels of strength, flexibility, energetic capacity, and integrity. Keep learning how you can move and open your body so that you don't contract, clam up, and grow old and feeble.

Growing Older, Smarter

As you age, you want to build your repertoire of anti-aging movement skills. Don't wait until you need to learn how to heal joints and strengthen your bones during an acute situation. Don't wait to build strength after a debilitating phase. Be proactive; start growing your skills and physical capacities now. Otherwise, at seventy, eighty, or ninety, you may end up in a body that is weak, lethargic, addicted, broken, run down, shrunken, fat, and unmotivated. By taking a proactive and experimental mindset, you learn as you go through each decade, broadening your body-optimization skill base and refining your self-healing capacities.

Get clear on where you lack body wisdom and need to fill in the gaps in your education. Get a coach to balance your weaknesses and train you to help yourself, heal yourself, and grow older, stronger, more flexible, more fit, and just plain smarter.

EXAMPLES OF BREATH-BODY PRACTICES

- Ten minutes stretching; ten minutes of exercises like jumping jacks, push-ups, or swinging a kettlebell

- Five minutes sitting pranayama, ten Sun Salutations, ten yoga standing poses

- Twenty-minute walk—swinging your arms, opening your joints—with deep conscious breathing

TIPS FOR YOUR BREATH-BODY HABIT

- Schedule it. Set your alarm. Get out any equipment the night before to keep your choices in line with what you want to have happen first thing the next day.

- As you fall asleep at night, visualize yourself doing the practice the next morning. See yourself going through the motions. You'll have less resistance the more you use visualization.

- Start at the same time, in the same place every day.

- After hydrating and pooping, go right to breath-centered movement. Don't delay or you risk distraction.

- A daily, twenty-minute practice is exponentially better than a two-hour practice twice a week. Longer isn't better. Shoot for consistency.

- Set goals for yourself and track your progress. Plan your workouts and fitness routines a week in advance.

- Go with what appeals to you right now.

- Or do the opposite if you've been in a rut or on a streak.

- Make sure you're well rested before increasing your exercise intensity. If you're not well rested, walk instead of working out.

- Vary the type of exercise between hardening, softening, and cardio, and vary the intensity of your workouts between challenging, moderate, and easy.

- Research what else is going on. If you've been doing yoga for a while, do some challenging bodyweight or strength training and vice versa. Expand your repertoire of movements, fitness, skills, and healing exercises so that you become more body-adept as you age.

- Find a coach or a teacher to inspire, guide, and train you.

HABIT 5

Fuel Yourself with a Plant-Based Diet

WHAT TO DO

If you want to be nourished deeply and receive abundance, tap into the consciousness of plants. Receive their gifts, and give back your care for their protection. Reenter the web of give and take. Shift from consumerism to collaboration. Feast upon higher quality phytonutrients, the raw material of your inner universe, through eating an increasingly diverse plant-based diet. You'll elevate your immune function and get connected to your local ecosystem or indoor gardening possibilities.

WHY YOU WANT TO DO IT

Deep nourishment is essential to light up your sensitive biochemistry. Poor nourishment leads your mind and emotions from discontent to despair and your body from lethargy to disrepair. Step up your nourish-to-flourish habits. When you connect your inner ecosystem (body) to your outer ecosystem (environment) through eating a local or regional diet, you develop a more grounded and interconnected presence and a stronger immune system.

You become a boon to the plants in your hood as your
sense of self extends to your ecosystem.

HOW TO START

Notice which vegetables and fruits you're attracted to when
you walk into your grocery store. Take them home with you.
Eat them. (Watch a YouTube video on how to prepare them.)
Diversify the plants in your diet to get more nutrition and
experience more energy. Also, learn about one edible plant
that grows in your yard or your hood—dandelions count.
Include your local food in your regular diet.

By now in the Body Thrive process, you should be metamorphosing.
You're establishing a higher standard for yourself. If you're on track, you're
experiencing a new playing field for how good you can feel, and you
know it'll just get better. At this altitude, your cravings are falling in line
with nature's wisdom. You don't enjoy what sinks your ship. You notice
you suffer more when you eat heavier later in the evening or skip your
morning movement. The habits are clicking in. And, if they are not, keep
reading and rereading the book. Find the power of the posse. The habits
will click in. Now we'll turn our attention to food. Yum.

Deep nourishment is what your body needs to thrive. Let's review
the core wisdom on how to receive nourishment. When you connect
with the plant, and the part of the life cycle it's in, you intuit the
plant's energy, wisdom, and nourishment. If you adulterate the plant,
its seed, or its soil, you miss out on a deeper experience of connectivity
on a soul level and on a deeper nourishment for your body.

What does deeper nourishment feel like? In a word, deep nourishment
feels good. Actually, it feels intrinsically abundant. You are supported by
the abundance of plants that are quick to grow and feed you. You borrow
their energy for the great purpose of your life or the subtle dharma of
your day. You give back and protect the plants as if they were your own
body, because indeed, they are. Until you are of this mindset, you will

feel subtly separate, disconnected, and not intrinsically nourished. Katrina Blair, author of one of my favorite books, *The Wild Wisdom of Weeds: 13 Essential Plants for Human Survival*, tells it like it is:

> The plant makes up our bones, skin, and cellular structure. The plant's essence infuses with our mind/heart. The plant's rooted intelligence from outside in the weather; under the sun, moon and stars; connected to the soil ecology; and tied intimately to the water of the land merges with our consciousness—creating an expansive sense of ourselves. By accepting that we need each other in respectful appreciation, the cycle of life sustains itself. This is the sacred act of reciprocal appropriation.[1]

Like a baby suckling at her mama's breast—eyes half closed, body relaxed—deep nourishment for grown-ups feels very much the same. You receive first, and then you give back. In the process, you experience wholeness, reciprocity, connectivity, and abundance. Your most fundamental relationship is your relationship with food, which mirrors your relationship with your body. If you are in dynamic cooperation with the plants that sustain you, you experience dynamic cooperation within yourself.

On a more analytical note about what you should eat, the data are in. The article "Nutritional Update for Physicians," published in *The Permanente Journal*, states:

> Research shows that plant-based diets are cost-effective, low-risk interventions that may lower body mass index, blood pressure, HbA1C, and cholesterol levels. They may also reduce the number of medications needed to treat chronic diseases and lower ischemic heart disease mortality rates. Physicians should consider recommending a plant-based diet to all their patients, especially those with high blood pressure, diabetes, cardiovascular disease, or obesity.[2]

Don't we all want to avoid high blood pressure, diabetes, cardiovascular disease, and obesity? The opposite of these diseases of stagnation is a clean, oxygenated, blood-pumping system; balanced endocrine function; optimal body weight; and a strong healthy heart. Our primate ancestors thrived on plants without falling prey to these diseases. Let's check out why.

Unlike most diets, a plant-based diet is defined by what it focuses on, not what it excludes. You maximize consumption of nutrient-dense plant foods while minimizing processed foods, oils, and animal foods. It's based on lots of vegetables (raw, fermented, roasted, cooked, boiled, char-broiled), fruits, beans, peas, lentils, seeds, and nuts (in smaller amounts).

Whether you include locally raised eggs, organic animal flesh, or bone broths is not worth getting worked into an analytical, left-brained tizzy. Honor your body by eating the whole foods it wants. Prioritize plants, which will detox your palate and create healthier cravings. If you eat animals, make sure they eat natural, local diets instead of imported fillers laced with hormones and antibiotics. Make sure they aren't tortured in how they are raised before slaughter. Their life becomes your bodily tissue, your emotions, and thought patterns. Enjoy a diet with loads of greens, stalks, and nonstarchy tubers, with fruits, legumes, grains, and seeds as well. You don't need to make strict rules about the meat, the wheat, the dairy, or sugars, unless you do so for ethical reasons, because you know these foods disrupt your system, or because you're in poor health and should experiment with an elimination diet. Either way, focus on plants becoming the star of your show.

Let's take the plant-based diet conversation to the next level and look at how nature is trying to feed us today, species and nutrient diversification, nutrient-dense superfoods, and our cravings.

More Plants in Your Diet

Experiment with your body to notice what makes you thrive. For me, after fifteen-plus years of experimenting with various detoxes and diets, I'm rendered with an absurd appetite for local wild weeds. My daily nutrification begins with a smoothie or green juice made from local native or invasive greens. If I'm quite hungry, I'll indulge in a living porridge: some soaked seeds (chia, flax, or sprouted almonds) and sprouted buckwheat mixed with cinnamon, raisins, maple syrup, and almond milk.

For lunch and dinner, I'll make a salad or a combo of leaves, shoots, and roots as the base of my meal, with room for beans, grains, or animal parts. (Call it what it is, right?) If it's cold or I have a hectic schedule or low energy, I'll opt for soup over salad, lightly cooked over raw.

Remember, the more complex or hard to digest your diet is, the less energy you have for everything else. Get good at streamlining your diet to optimize your energy. Food on a daily basis should be more simple than fancy, more nourishing than disruptive to your body balance.

The following chart offers some ideas for keeping food simple. (You'll find recipes at bodythrive.com/free.)

Breakfast Ideas

Green juice or smoothie (celery, cucumbers, alfalfa sprouts, supergreen powder mix, dandelion greens, and fresh fruit)

Chia porridge with sprouted buckwheat granola and almond milk

Stewed apples with spices

Oatmeal with raisins and soaked almonds

Miso soup and pickled vegetables (Asian breakfast)

Chard and eggs

Lunch Ideas

Green salad with white beans

Roasted beets, sautéed green beans, and goat cheese

Lentil and vegetable soup

Kale salad with avocado and pine nuts

Acorn squash baked with brussels sprouts

Caesar salad with chicken

Dinner Ideas

Curried carrot-coconut soup

French onion soup

Kitchari (rice and mung-bean stew)

Chicken vegetable soup

A hummus and crudités plate

Ceviche on a bed of local greens

I don't spend much time in the kitchen. Yet I prepare 90 percent of what I eat. I love my diet and have a strong connection with the plants I eat. What is abundant and seasonal is regional, so I don't often venture into complex concoctions or store-bought prepared foods. The bonus chapter at the end of the book, Kitchen Sadhana, explains how.

Plants and the Gifting Economy

Eating a plant-based diet is not really about what to eat and what not to eat. Plants feed us directly or indirectly through the animals in our diet. A plant-based diet is about awakening to our shared and intelligent ecology. It's about receiving plant wisdom, consciousness, and nutrition on a cellular, as well as a spiritual, level.

When we feel a conscious connection to the plants we rely on, we feel gifted, abundant, and truly nourished. With this connection comes the realization that we are continually being gifted with the sunlight, the air, the soil, the water, the plants, the earth, the trees. Indebted to the gifts that sustain us, we reciprocate by offering our protection and cooperation. In return, we desire to leave the planet and the world better off from our being here. Completing the cycle, we elevate the game. Our desires, ideas, and actions confirm our interconnection and giftedness.

As we feel grateful and our sense of self expands, our care expands with it. Our compulsion is to pay it forward, to give ourselves fully back to the web of life and impulse of evolution. I'm giving the mic back to resident expert here on Planet Earth, author Katrina Blair:

> Trends in nature predominantly focus on paying it forward. The resources build up and become available over time. The gifting economy in human societies works when we each focus on doing what we love. The energy and joy that comes from spending time focusing our natural talents becomes a gift and act of service to others. When we engage in activities that have authentic meaning for us, we enter into the river of a gifting economy.

All beings have a sacred purpose on Earth, and we engage in a noble contract when we experience life's give and take as a dance of sacred interconnectedness.[3]

Plants humble us by filling our nutrient neediness with their generosity. As our orientation to life evolves through connection to the plants and the planet, we feel intrinsic fullness within our biochemistry. It's the same intrinsic experience of fullness, connectivity, and abundance expressed by the word *purnatva* that the yogis talk about. It enables us to become a helpful, contributing component within our ecosystem and communities. The less we adulterate the plant we are eating, including its genetic chemistry or how we process it, the more life energy, nutrients, and wisdom we receive directly from that plant.

One of the ways to tap into purnatva via plants is to eat more species of plants. When you diversify the plants you eat, you receive a broader base of nutrition for your cells. Complexity in nutrients leads to cellular nutrition. Biodiversity is healthy and begins at home, in your body.

Evolve from Consumer to Collaborator

Just as each friend you have is different from the rest, each plant species in your diet becomes a new friend. Yet 75 percent of what humans eat today is generated by twelve plants and five animal species. Ouch. Of the 250,000 to 300,000 known edible plant species, only 150 to 200 are used by humans. Three plants—rice, maize, and wheat—contribute nearly 60 percent of calories and proteins obtained by humans from plants. The Food and Agriculture Organization of the United Nations estimates that during the last century, 75 percent of crop genetic diversity has been lost, a phenomenon referred to as *genetic erosion*, as farmers worldwide have opted for (or been coerced into) planting genetically uniform high-yield seeds, using petrochemicals, and monocropping.[4]

That means that global industry and industrial agriculture have killed 75 percent of our agrobiodiversity in less than a hundred years. Holy disaster, Batman! And we haven't just lost the plants; we've lost a huge chunk of our bioculture: our local food-production systems including local knowledge and the culture, skills, and even languages of women and men farmers. Not just harvested seeds are disappearing, but also unharvested species that we don't know much about. It's as if our planet is losing part of its brain to monocultured junk food, which is echoed in this quote from *Sustainability* magazine:

> Genetic erosion is linked to cultural erosion—and the loss of seeds linked to the loss of human culture or languages globally. Indeed, cultures are diminishing like the seeds of so many plants. Linguists, for example, indicate that 60 to 90 percent of the world's 6,800 languages will be extinguished by the end of the century.[5]

With the loss of species and languages, we have also lost deep wisdom in how to prepare great food. How is genetic and cultural erosion happening so quickly? We have shifted from dynamic ecosystem collaborators to mainstream consumers. More people ask me, "What should I eat?" instead of, "What should I do today to care for my ecosystem?" It's grievous how far down the path to consumer mentality we've come in just a hundred years.

If you want more control over what you're eating, you need to get more involved with plants and farms. We must shift, one by one, from consumer to collaborator. The good news is that it's really fun. The first step is to turn back to variety, the spice of life. Nature is trying to nourish you. Expand your horizons.

What Is Palatable to Your Palate?

What we like to eat is relative. Our palates have forgotten the unique flavors of the plant friends our ancestors loved. What is palatable changes with what we feed ourselves. Our cravings may be predictable, but they are not fixed. As you get older, if your body wisdom grows, your cravings get smarter. You become more sensitive and aware of which plants or animals are noticeably nourishing.

The inverse is just as true. As you age, if your body wisdom stagnates, your cravings get dumber. You feed yourself based on cravings, which recycle physical or emotional addictions and uninformed habits. Your unintelligent cravings deplete, poison, and destroy you slowly, one sip or bite at a time, from the inside out.

I've led thousands of people through Ayurvedic detoxes since I founded the Yogidetox program in 2002. The most predictable outcomes reported by Yogidetoxers are the release of excess weight, improvement of sleep, and the overall feeling of falling in love with one's life. Yet what surprises Yogidetoxers the most is that as their desires get smarter, their addictions fall away. Repeatedly, they say:

- I don't crave baked goods.

- I'm no longer wanting a glass of wine with dinner.

- I don't want _____ anymore. (bread, coffee, beer, cheese, meat, chips, ice cream, pizza, etc.)

The cruel paradox is that if your cravings are dumb, they make you dumber. Taste is relative to what you've relished recently. What you crave is almost always determined by the pattern you are in. If you've been eating cookies every day, you will crave cookies. If you've been adding lemon to your water every day, you will crave lemon-water tomorrow. Like increases like, and the opposites reduce each other. When you start to diversify the species in your diet to diversify the nutrients, what is palatable to you expands. When you eat seasonally, you crave what is in season. Because you can change what you crave, be smart when designing tomorrow's cravings.

Refresher on Plant Parts as Food

The different parts and stages of plants reflect and enable us to connect with the cycles of life itself. The lifecycle of plants goes like this: seed, sprout, root, stalk, leaf, flower, fruit, and back to seed.

Are seeds better than sprouts? Are roots better than stalks? Ridiculous, right? All parts serve a purpose. All plants bear a gift. Refer to the table on the next page for a refresher.

Physical Body	Mental and Emotional Body	Examples
Oil, fat, deep nutrients, deep energy—builds body tissue	Provides grounding and a heavy, potent energy; most seeds need to be soaked or roasted first.	Spice seeds, grain and legume seeds, nuts, oil seeds, anything that can sprout
Quick energy, protein, boatloads of nutrients	Zippy, energized, childlike, quick energy	Alfalfa sprouts, sunflower sprouts, bean sprouts, sprouted quinoa
Minerals, fiber; sugars	Building energy, grounding, nutrifying; balance with leaves to avoid stagnation	Carrots, beets, potatoes, radishes, yams, jicama
Hydration, fiber, low calorie, great for chewing the cud without calories	The chewing action relaxes the jaw and the nervous system	Celery, broccoli stalks, chard stalks, dandelion stems, kale stalks
Sunlight energy, chlorophyll, nutrients, minerals, cleansing, scraping, and contracting; boatloads of nutrients	Quick daily energy, clarifying, cleansing, removes stagnation	Lettuces, kale, collards, dandelion greens
Nurtures the senses and soul	Adds beauty, sensitivity, refinement, and joy	Roses, Johnny jump-ups, lavender, fennel
Sugars, quick carbs, replenishes blood sugar energy quickly	The sweet, heavy quality of fruit creates relaxation and ease, reminding us of the sweetness of life	Apples, bananas, avocados, pineapples, dates, raisins, grapes

Evolve Your Cells with Nutrient Diversity

The more diverse the nutrient complex of your diet, the more building blocks your body has to build sound tissue. If the name of the game is a high-nutrient, mostly regional diet, where do we find high-nutrient foods? There is a scare in our culture about food-nutrient depletion. Our topsoil is depleted. Many of our plants are now engineered. Our soil, our plants, and therefore our food aren't what they used to be. Most of our meat is deranged through factory farming. We aren't getting the nutrients our bodies want out of the foods in our grocery stores.

At the same time, natural grocers are opening new aisles filled with imported superfoods—goji berries, maca, acai berry, chia, spirulina, dehydrated coconut crystals, quinoa, amaranth, chlorella and a zillion other green powders, reishi, bee pollen, camu camu berry, hemp, cacao, hijiki. Our options and our taste buds are expanding quickly. The medicinal and supplement section of the grocery store overflows with plants from around the world packed in bottles. This is excellent—and problematic.

Superfoods are packaged and sold as expensive designer nutrients to affluent, educated health-seekers. Most superfoods are harvested far from the ecosystems where they are consumed. The connection between caretaker of that ecosystem and consumer is broken, and the nutrient-dense plants become premium priced on the global market. The locals of that ecosystem can no longer afford the superfoods, as exemplified by the rising cost of quinoa for Peruvians. Therefore, while the superfoods are indeed super, they don't tap the origin of the issue or solve all of our problems.

What is a Body Thriver to do? Look to nature for the solution. Nature provides solutions, inviting us to observe, cooperate, and integrate. Now, for a wider perspective on how nature is trying to feed us, we'll take a walk on the wild side.

Have No Fear, the Invasive Weeds Are Here

Many of the next generation of superfoods will be our hyper-prolific, biodynamic, permaculture, common invasive weeds. We have barely tapped the natural productivity of our regional ecosystem potential.

Nutrients that can protect our immune systems grow in our own backyard regional ecosystems. Our shared planetary invasive superfoods are everywhere you want to be. Yet most of us don't know that invasives can nourish our bodies as easily, if not better, than the pricey, hip, imported superfoods.

The invasive species—dandelion, thistle, lamb's quarters, miner's lettuce, stinging nettle, burdock, mullein, and purslane—have taken residence in your region. They pop up and thrive where soil is disturbed due to their ecological competence. They are succession plants, thriving in the harshest of conditions that humans inflict on the earth's sensitive topsoil.

The invasives are impossible to eradicate even with chemical warfare, which in turn renders topsoil and neighborhoods horrifically toxic. Of course, chemical warfare on weeds ends up in groundwater and in our bodies. What goes around, comes around. The invasives are barely affected and continue to overtake native species planet-round, further altering the familiar landscape.

But this doesn't need to be a bad, sad story. Like Roman emperor Marcus Aurelius wrote millennia ago, "The impediment to action advances action. What stands in the way becomes the way."

Invasives grow roots so strong and so deep that they break through concrete to grab nutrients from the deep earth. Their dharma is to refertilize and remineralize the soil we have wrecked, and then move on. Some have tap-roots ten to sixty feet deep to access nutrients, minerals, and vitamins below the disturbed topsoil and bring them up to the surface. The wild invasives are superconductors, pulling water and micronutrients through the crust, deep beneath our destroyed topsoil—the barrier our kale and carrots can't penetrate—and bringing the nutrients up through their shoots, into their leaves, flowers, and fruits.[6] The wild invasives are here to save our day, to become both our garden and our medicine cabinet.

Backyard invasive nutrients offer their immune resilience to your immune resilience. When you eat plants that thrive in your ecosystem, you borrow their local intelligence. When you eat the plants that thrive in your ecosystem, they lend you their thrive. If you eat the wild invasive weeds in your yard and you blend the tender dandelion and young thistle leaves into your morning green smoothie, you *become* your local ecosystem. If you don't eat your local plant friends, you eventually become allergic to your local ecosystem.

When you first start eating wild plants or wild weeds, you notice they taste *wild*. You will find them not as palatable as their domesticated brethren in the grocery store. You can taste the raw elements and exotic phytonutrients in them. You can taste the wildness, prana, and plant chemistry in their natural state. You are eating the foods more nutritionally akin to what your ancient ancestors ate, which awakens both your informed ancestral memory and primal energy.

The most common reaction to eating local, wild weeds and native plants is to be alarmed at their intensity. They have intense flavors and wild energies. Our palates are domesticated, emasculated, castrated, if you will, and cut off from real nutrients. But remember, tastes are acquired: taste is relative to what you've relished recently.

As my palate wised up, I wanted to know the native edibles in my ecosystem. As I learned, I planted them in my yard. When I heard a botanist say that thistle, a prickly beast of a plant, was edible, I did some research and experimented. Over time, my garden played second fiddle as I harvested the thistle, dandelion, lamb's quarters, amaranth, miner's lettuce, and alfalfa volunteers. Even young thistle leaves mix nicely in a high-speed blender with apples, a squeeze of lemon, a sprig of mint, and water. The prickles turn silky smooth in a green smoothie. The taste? Wild.

I'll keep saying it: wild foods taste wild. You can't expect your conditioned, domesticated, globally imported palate to embrace the wild landscape. You are going back one to two hundred years, tasting minerals and micronutrients you've never tasted. Yet, after you condition your palate to wild foods, you crave them. Like increases like. Repetition cultures your habits. The more you dig dandelion and thistle, the more you dig dandelion and thistle. The next thing you know, you'll be sporting a message on your T-shirt that says, "Dandelions are the new kale" or "Thistle is the new dandelion."

Navigating the Urban Landscape

I realize not all of you have a thistle patch in your yard. Many of you are urban and are not about to pluck the invasive purslane growing in the sidewalk cracks and throw it in your blender.

Leaving wild foods aside, let's back up a step and focus on species diversification. When you diversify the plants in your diet, you diversify the nutrients in your body. As you connect with the plants and imbibe the diversity of nutrients, you will have the experience that nature is trying its damnedest to take care of you. With that orientation, you enter thrive.

If you live in a city, hopefully you're going to the farmers markets weekly in season. Hopefully you are growing a few plants in your kitchen and sprouting seeds on your counter. You can grow greens year-round through windowsill gardening. If you don't know how, listen to the "Indoor Gardening" episode on the Yogahealer podcast.

If you live in a city, you probably feel more like a consumer, so it's important for your psyche to take action to enter the collaborative cycle. Your demand is much of what is driving today's economic landscape. Spread the word. Take a stand against Roundup-ready yards. Educate yourself and your peers. Be a dynamic conversationalist. Evolve from consumer to collaborator.

At the farmers market, get in touch with the market value of nutrient-dense food in your region and know the price; it's a good value for your body and spirit. Add plants with the colors and textures that grab your attention. Experiment with flavors to stimulate your palate. Talk to your region's farmers about why they farm. Ask if they'll start to truck their edible weeds to town along with their domesticated plants. Tell them that together you can raise demand and make their work easier. Wild weeds grow themselves! The farmers have to weed them out anyway, so they might as well load them in the truck. Due to demand, you can now easily find dandelion greens, lamb's quarters, and purslane in grocery stores. I hope Whole Foods's "365" label or Jamba Juice will offer a local, invasive, green-food powder. What you want and who you express your desire to matters.

You can't trade your butter lettuce for thistle overnight. With "yes, and," you don't have to. Though you may already have a great diet, ask yourself, "And what can I add?" To start to track in the categories from nonlocal to local invasives, make a simple chart, and use a rating system to track and keep score: nonlocal plants count for 1; regional plants count for 2; local, wild, edible plants count for 3; invasives count for 4.

Paleo(lithic) Diet: The Pre-Agriculture Approach

I love the paleo diet. Except for the prejudice against sweet, juicy fruits; beans; and grains. Oh, and the common practice of eating animal flesh or organs two to three times a day. No, really, I do love paleo, except for those things. Here is why:

- The idea of paleo is based on the plants that primitive humans ate.

- Processed food is out. High-glycemic and carbohydrate fillers are out.

- You're acting more like a cave(wo)man, eating mostly leafy greens, shoots, roots, nuts, and seeds.

- You can simplify your food preparation.

- The paleo people of today are connected and enthusiastic. They can help spread the word about edible invasives, and they'll be behind our Roundup-Ready Removal Revolution.

So, if you're going paleo, go paleo-*invasivor*. "Invasivorism is the act of eating invasive species, on purpose, in order to lower their numbers," says Joe Roman, conservation biologist and founder of eattheinvaders.org.[7] Joe defines *invasivorism* as "directing our appetite in a way that could have a positive impact." His plan is pure, awake, connected genius. If you eat fish, eat carp (an invasive species), not the endangered swordfish. In some places in the United States, feral pigs are a problem, so if you eat pork, why not eat feral pigs that have been hunted in the area? When you eat invasives, you nourish yourself with what the ecosystem is providing in excess. You help both the ecosystem and your body to thrive as nature intended.

Let's not forget the underlying message from both Ayurveda and the plant-based diet: get to know yourself. Experiment. What works for you? Be honest. Not everyone is grain- or gluten- or dairy- or legume-intolerant. Not everyone needs animal parts, but some people do. Make your choices according to your own discoveries. Honor your ethics for sustainable, diverse nutrition for all. Become a dynamic collaborator with our planetary ecosystem.

TIPS FOR A PLANT-BASED DIET

- Track the species you eat and add a new species every week or month.

- Favor nutrient-dense foods.

- Become aware of the phase in the cycle of the food on your plate. Diversify your diet to eat roots and leaves (greens), fruits, and seeds. Start with awareness.

- If you need to lose weight or smarten your cravings, join the next Yogidetox at yogidetox.com. You'll learn about acid-alkaline balance and how to eat detoxifying and healing foods on a regular basis.

- Eat leafy greens and nonstarchy roots. Limit starchy roots.

- Eat foods of every color of the rainbow. It's fun, and you get more phytonutrients.

- Learn which foods and edible weeds grow easily in your ecosystem.

- Find a local botanist and organize a local edible plant walk. This sounds harder than it is. People and plants will thank you for it.

- Read Katrina Blair's book *The Wild Wisdom of Weeds: 13 Essential Plants for Human Survival.*

- Listen for which plant foods call your name when you walk down the produce aisle. Put them in your cart. The prana in the plants is still alive and connecting with your prana. Honor that connection, and you'll gain more access into your intuitive body.

- Before eating, take time to pause and connect with the plants on your plate.

- Get your plant foods in season from a community supported agriculture (CSA) program or farmers market.

- Grow your own food, even if it's just sprouting sprouts and microgreens on your counter.

- Ask farmers at the market about buying their edible weeds. Talk to those you influence about increasing demand for edible invasives. Give them a good rap.

- If you eat meat or bone broths, find a regional CSA meat farm and stock your freezer. Get a small deep freezer if you need more space.

- Buy the eggs of heirloom chickens.

INTERLUDE

How to Evolve Your Habits in Relationships

Following the 10 Habits of Body Thrive leads to living life on your own terms, interdependently. As you dial in these habits, you're constructing the building blocks of a vibrant life. The Body Thrive Habits shift your identity. Take a moment to consider how your body is shape-shifting, how your thoughts are smarter, and how your emotions are more positive. The Body Thrive Habits will also clarify, change, and evolve your relationships. If you are integrating the habits in your daily life, you may notice that your relationships are also shifting.

My clients are often surprised when the core people in their lives aren't gung ho about evolving right alongside them. They get inspired and want to ignite the drive to evolve in others. Sometimes this happens, and their partner, kids, parents, and best friends are in for the ride. More often, they aren't.

The core people in your life may be happy just as they are and not interested in shape-shifting their diet and lifestyle alongside you. This can create a world of tension, discomfort, frustration, and depression as you come to terms with trying to move forward while feeling dragged back.

This section, which is a brief intermission from the Body Thrive Habits, is about navigating your core relationships as you evolve your habits. This chapter is filled with tools—from super-easy tactics to navigating sticky or stuck situations. Without these tools, you will get frustrated and your progress will be unnecessarily slow.

In addition to navigating your core relationships as you evolve your habits, another crucial piece is this: *you need to spend more time with people who have the daily habits you want.* Surround yourself with people you admire.

How to Ask for Support with Habit Evolution

As you are changing your habits, it's simply kind to inform others. Not only does that help you stay accountable to yourself by having others know, it also gives your people a heads up. The real boon here is that you can also deliberately and specifically ask for support.

In asking, we are humbled. We admit that we are interdependent, not isolated, and that we affect each other. Let me show you the simplest, most effective way I've found to mobilize support. And you'll be more likely to support others on their growth paths once you know this strategy. Follow these steps:

1. Determine the habit you want to have. Be specific. For example: go to bed by 9:00 p.m. or wake up and work out for twenty minutes before 7:30 a.m.

2. Determine who may influence your habits or be affected by them, consciously or unconsciously. Write your list, including people you live with, dependents, friends, colleagues, and influencers (educators, writers, bloggers, podcasters) whom you may follow.

3. Schedule a five-minute check-in. If you have access to the people who influence you, ask them if you could arrange a quick meeting with them about a habit you are trying to change. Schedule the meeting for a neutral time. You want their full attention; don't try to slip this into a casual conversation or throw it into an argument.

If you have children, you can schedule meetings with them too.

4. At the meeting, tell the person the "why" behind the habit you want to change. For example, Jasmine (whom you met in the Start Your Day Right chapter) told her partner, "I am really tired when I put the two-year-old to bed. My body just wants to be done with the day and go to sleep. This may sound wacky, but I want to start going to sleep then, or whenever my body signals it's done with the day."

5. Ask the person if they are willing to support you in this habit change. Often your change in habits affects other people. Be clear on what will be affected and how you want to manage those effects. In Jasmine's case, by going to sleep earlier, she couldn't help finish the dishes or laundry or connect in conversation with her husband. Once you know what's at stake for this habit to change—for all parties—you can ask for informed support.

6. Determine *specific* ways you want support. Giving support is absurdly easy when the other person knows exactly what they can do to help you. If necessary, brainstorm to figure out what that is. Asking for a specific, nonsnarky reminder is often the easiest and most effective way for your influencers to support you. I ask my husband to remind me that I'd rather have a raw ginger ball instead of whatever he is having for dessert. I ask him to remind me in an emotionally neutral way. Not teasing. Not cajoling. Just reminding me. You can use the trigger-habit-reward method around support.
   - Example of using an emotional trigger: "When you hear me talking too fast, will you remind me to take a deep breath?"
   - Example of using an activity trigger (note how you can also ask people not to offer you things

you are trying to consume less of): "If you're getting drinks, I'd like hot water with lemon. Please don't ask me if I want a glass of wine. That would be a tremendous help."

Jasmine asked her husband to support her new bedtime habit. He determined he would finish the dishes while she put the two-year-old and herself to bed. After a few check-ins, they decided to invest $50 per week in household services. They found a responsible high school student who could do light housework and play with the two-year-old for a few hours on the weekend while they took a hike with the baby. They got in their adult conversation. Jasmine began to get the sleep she needed.

After a few months of going to bed when her body first signaled fatigue in the evening, Jasmine woke up feeling rested. It took months. Eventually, she woke up wanting to breathe and move. Then her breath-body practice could move onto center stage, yet Go to Bed Early remained her keystone habit.

You can evolve your relationship habits and dynamics like any other habit change. Be creative. Experiment and take risks as you go along. See what works for you and your peeps. That is it. That is how you ask for support in your habit evolution.

How to Have Your Weekly Thrive Meeting

When you realize how easy it is to ask for and receive support, you may want to incorporate weekly thrive meetings. I recommend this for everyone—whether it's a weekly chat session with a good friend or a scheduled time to check in with your family or anyone you share space and live with.

At home, we have a quick family meeting at some point during the weekend. Usually it's a spontaneous affair after a weekend breakfast. However, as you're getting started with this, schedule a consistent time. The more people involved, the more time you need.

Set a time for a twenty-minute weekly meeting that will work for everyone. (I encourage kids of all ages to come; it will help them learn this basic skill!) Once you have a time established, put it on your schedule. Don't cancel without rescheduling. At your weekly meetings, here's what you should cover:

1. State why you are meeting. You can use this statement or come up with your own: "We are coming together for a short conversation to check in with each other, to find out how to support each other during the week ahead, and to resolve any issues that keep us from thriving together. Let's get started."

2. Give the talking stick to one person at a time, working through the following questions. Divide the amount of time you have by the number of people present so that no one dominates. Move through the list below with one person before going to the next.
   - What is going on for you this week? What are your goals for the week?
   - What worked well or didn't work for you last week?
   - How can any of us support you this week? Do you have any specific needs or requests? (Listen deeply.)
   - Do you want to clear the air about anything with anyone? (This is a call for grievances and an opportunity to clear the air.)

3. Switch to the next person.

With practice, the meetings are quick. Don't use this time to dispute complicated issues or do co-counseling. If someone needs more time, schedule a session just for them. If this happens repeatedly, ask that person to listen more than speak—for the harmony of the whole group.

In the beginning, new habits are awkward. You can't expect asking for support and having a weekly meeting to be anything but awkward at first. However, if you commit to it, you'll find that you fly through the meeting and that the days between meetings enhance cooperation and goodwill.

The weekly meeting works for best friends, couples, and families as much as it does for companies or mastermind groups. Schedule it in. Ask yourself, "How easy can it be?" Show up and stick to the agenda. Bring a positive attitude, your care for others, open expectations, and a bucket of curiosity.

What If Your People Don't Want to Evolve?

I used to look for support in all the wrong places. I wanted my husband to be as excited and motivated about diet and lifestyle evolution as I was. I wanted my dad to coach me in my career because he had been a successful businessman. I wanted my old friends to become thought leaders and community catalysts. I wanted all sorts of things from all sorts of people who were more interested in other pursuits. Instead of replacing all my key relationships—parents, husband, siblings, friends—I decided to notice what these folks were already bringing to the table.

See the choice point there? To decide is to put something to death—think pesti*cide*, homi*cide*, sui*cide*, infanti*cide*. When you decide, you put to death the other options so you can redirect your attention toward what you want to grow. I put to death the idea of receiving specific support where it didn't already exist in order to redirect my attention to where I could easily receive that specific support. I decided not to expect or even ask my peeps for gifts they could not easily give. This was a tremendous breakthrough for me. Prior to my "aha" moment, I had all sorts of expectations. Not only was I unrighteously disappointed, I wasn't getting my needs met. So instead, I decided to consciously receive the gifts they were already giving.

Then I made a pivotal decision. I decided to seek how I could actually find the specific support I wanted in my career. I searched and found new social circles. I looked for and found great business coaches. I discovered brilliant collaborators and accountability partners on the same path. I formed mastermind groups with colleagues more determined and skilled in the arenas I wanted to pursue. I hired coaches who were more organized, efficient, and accomplished than myself. I stopped looking for support where it didn't exist.

Relationship Agreements

The path of Body Thrive leads to an awake life. As your body thrives at a higher vibration, your care expands, your ideas are more interconnected, and you want to grow in all aspects of your life: health, career, relationships, finances, personal integrity, dharma, philanthropy.

When you're growing at an accelerated rate, you may feel like you're surrounded by sticks-in-the-mud. You'll find many of your friends or family members have beliefs you no longer hold. You may want to break away from victim mentality, complacency, and complaining. A T-shirt from a microbrewery in Bozeman, Montana, comes to mind: "No Whiners" was their motto.

Many of my clients realize that they are partnered with addicts. They wake up to their own addictions and enabling behavior. Their partner's habit of daily drug or alcohol consumption, junk food, overeating, television, workaholism, or whatever the addictive pattern may be isn't what they want to do anymore. At first, they might try to motivate change in others. Then, if change isn't happening, they need to update their relationship agreements in those core relationships.

The agreements in our core relationships are either outdated or updated. If the agreements are not articulated, they can quickly become outdated. If you're operating on outdated, unspoken agreements, the relationship isn't as dynamic, inspired, evolutionary, supportive, or connective as you want it to be on the Body Thrive path. Take the time to step back and consciously update your relationship agreements to line up with your potential.

How to Uplevel Your Relationship Agreements

You'll find the relationship agreement conversation below very similar to the weekly meeting, except that it doesn't happen weekly and you can go much deeper.

Schedule a neutral time for a sixty- to ninety-minute conversation. It might actually be much shorter. You might start the meeting saying something like this: "We are meeting to become aware of (or refresh) the agreements we have in our relationship. We will check in with each other to find out how to support each other's growth, to clear the air as necessary, and to resolve any unspoken issues that keep us from growing. Let us begin." Then, take turns discussing the following:

- What are the growing edges in your life right now?

- What do you want from our relationship?

- Are there any outdated agreements or unresolved issues between us?

- I'm interested in supporting your growth. Let's explore a few specific ways I can support you.

- Let's name ethics and shared values our relationship is now based on.

These questions are guidelines. Find questions that work for you to update your relationships in line with where you want to go and help you to help others.

Core Relationship Scenarios around Habit Evolution

Over my years of leading Yogidetox groups and Body Thrive coaching, I've seen two basic relationship scenarios play out when one person starts to make the Body Thrive changes.

Scenario A goes like this: Thistley, who has always been into yoga, goes on a serious health kick with Ayurveda. She detoxes, turning herself and her kitchen upside down and inside out. She buys an expensive blender or juicer. She starts doing self-massage and going to bed early. She starts meditating before dawn. The spare tire around her middle shrinks, leaving a lovely waistline. Her inner gorgeousness shines through brighter than it has in years. She is tapping into her inner beauty—fueled with deep body wisdom and devoted to evolving her habits over the long haul. Soon her partner is also asking for a green smoothie. Because it's not much fun staying up late alone, her partner starts turning in earlier. Because Thistley doesn't drink much at night anymore, they take walks or do household projects after dinner. Thistley is meeting new friends at yoga class who have healthier, inspiring relationships. Their social circle transforms to match their higher vibration. (The tools in this chapter facilitate this type of scenario.)

Scenario B goes like this: Dandi, who has always been into yoga, goes on a serious health kick with Ayurveda. She detoxes and turns her kitchen upside down and inside out. She buys an expensive blender or juicer. She starts doing self-massage, going to bed early, waking up early, and meditating. Her spare tire falls off. Her inner gorgeousness shines through brighter than it has in years. You know the story.

In this scenario, Dandi's partner complains that she isn't as fun as she used to be. She's too serious now. She doesn't want to go out and share a bottle of wine. She is less interested in sex because she is not attracted to him. Dandi and her partner drift apart, each preferring to spend time with people who are on their wavelength. They stay together, living separate lives like roommates under a legal or religious contract, but in a field of negative tension. Or, they split.

I routinely witness scenario A, B, or something in-between as people navigate habit evolution. If you find yourself somewhere on this spectrum, know you are not alone. And while this period may not be easy, set your sights—and your habits—on the life you desire. Start by looking for support in all the right places.

Look for Support in All the Right Places

I have a simple tool that can help you orient yourself toward growth relationships. Start here. Make a chart. Fill in the columns with names of the core people in your life.

Your Uplifters, Champions, and Upholders	The Middlers	The Backsliders

1. The first column is people who bolster your potential. They hold you to a level of integrity you strive for in yourself. These people uphold you to be all that you can be. They don't let you slide. They champion you.

2. The middle column is people who do let you slide some of the time. They themselves may not have clear relationship agreements. They sometimes inspire and sometimes

challenge you, but often are comfortable company and don't hold you to your higher standard.

3. The third column is for people who are victim oriented, pessimistic, and undermine their own and your growth. You may have once related and connected with these people, but now you find yourself uninterested and uninspired by the conversation. At times you may wake up to the fact that you are no longer wanting to plug into certain relationships.

Now that you have your chart, you may have realized a few things. You may have an overflowing column or an empty column. Hopefully, your chart is weighted to the left, not the right. In any case, this is what you want to do next:

1. Focus on your Uplifters, Champions, and Upholders, if you have any. Schedule a time to talk. Let them know you value your relationship and want to take a little time to get clear on how you can support each other. Make an informal (or formal) agreement based on holding you to a level of integrity you strive for in yourself.

2. With the Middlers list, ask if they are interested in making an informal or formal relationship agreement based on holding you to a level of integrity you strive for in yourself. They might not get it at first but will probably find the conversation insightful.

3. In the Backsliders column: If there is a core person in your life who you feel doesn't support you or understand where you're at, you need to schedule a relationship-agreement conversation. This will create clarity and a new platform for both of you. And remember, people can jump columns at any time, especially when you invite them to step into integrity with support.

You may have a sense it will take time to update your relationship agreements and navigate toward those who are inspiring—who breathe life into you. This simple tool does take time and accountability. Create circumstances where you can be influenced by those who are hitting the mark rather than those who are missing the mark. You may be a terrific inspiration to those in the Backslider column over time.

When you're growing, shifting, and evolving, you want to stabilize your growth. You don't want to backslide. You need to know who is on your Champions list. You need to know where to turn for the best advice. You need to know whom you want to be influenced by, because we all influence each other all the time. Next, let's look at consciously creating your tribe.

Build Your Tribe

When I was teaching this concept to my Yogidetox students years ago, I told them to look at the "Favorites" in their cell phone. I asked them to see how it matched up with looking for support in all the right places.

A key to habit evolution is evolutionary peer support. In yoga we call this *kula*, or "community of the heart." In Buddhism, we call it *sangha*, or "community of practitioners." In behavioral science, we call it "peer support."

For your foundling habits, you need to take the peer support ultra-seriously. Blow off this part, and no, you won't shoot yourself in the foot again: you'll simply be binding your feet. Without peer support, you can only take baby steps like those cruelly mistreated Chinese women from past eras. Why take baby steps when the mother of all mothers is granting you giant steps?

If the words *peer support* don't work for you, try the word *tribe*, a first-chakra word meaning where you are rooted. *Tribe* is your people, your base, an extension of yourself. The people you surround yourself with become who you are. When you're evolving your habits, I recommend finding or forming a tribe—a community of the heart—that already has that habit in motion.

For instance, let's take the meditation habit, which we'll be diving into shortly. I know more students have struggled to get the meditation habit dialed into a daily routine than any other actionable habit listed here. Meditation, or the sitting-in-silence habit, may seem out of reach in an overstimulated, exciting, rapidly evolving world unfolding in the big mystery. To sit in silence may be arduous at first. If we can't make arduous into easy, we'll fail.

What if you called in the troops—the tribe? There are already groups of people meditating, locally or online. Get yourself in the middle of guidance and support. You can join one of the many free, online meditation communities, like Craig Hamilton's. Or join a Body Thrive Coaching group and connect with a coach and a posse of people just like you who want to create their new normal.

Find an Accountability Partner

Let's take another habit: Go to Bed Early. Let's say everyone in your household goes to bed late. You're the only one interested in changing your bedtime. Obviously, you can't ditch this tribe. But ask around. Let your friends know you're trying to go to bed earlier. See if anyone else has that habit. See if anyone else wants to work on that habit, in earnest, right now.

When you find someone who has that habit or wants that habit, create an accountability partnership. While only you can really hold yourself accountable, having someone to check in with and reflect back to you can make you much more accountable to yourself.

With a partner, you could have a five-minute morning check-in: "Did you go to bed by your 10:00 p.m. goal? No? What choices will you make today to ensure you're on target for an earlier bedtime tonight?" Or, if this habit is too challenging, pull a kaizen move and ask, "How can you make the habit easier?" Or, if your partner is repeatedly failing, despite kaizen and multiple suggestions, return to their big "why." Is their big "why" big enough?

If you want an accountability partner, go to the Yogahealer Facebook page and put it out there. A post like this will work just fine: "Non-meditator seeking meditator who loves their practice to be my accountability partner for two months. I'll help hold you account-able for your positive self-improvement goal. Message me."

The beauty of now is the interconnectivity of the Internet. Tribes who have all these habits are inviting you to join them. In the Yogahealer online courses, I encourage my students to pair with an accountability partner. Some work on Body Thrive goals; others focus on business, career, or freedom lifestyle goals. If you're looking for a community and it doesn't exist locally or isn't quite what you're looking for, go online. Find a website or two that exude the skill or habit you wish you had. Sign up for their free training or mailing list. Learn from their blog, podcast, or videos. Find a community that inspires and delights you.

Then sign up for a program, a course, a class, or a coach. When you have skin in the game, you are more dedicated to the outcome.

The Company You Keep

You've probably heard statements like "You are the average of the five people you spend the most time with" from the late motivational speaker Jim Rohn. Other sayings are popular too: "You become the company you keep, so keep great company," and "Keep good company. Company makes a man great."

Most of my clients are women, and most people reading this book will be women. Women, being higher in the water element according to Ayurveda, morph more easily than men. You can see this in our higher body-fat ratio coupled with the morphology of having babies. Women tend to morph into what is needed of them or as a result of the current situation. Our flow is a blessing for others, and can be a curse for us. Many of my clients on the growth path find that their relationships don't serve who they are becoming and pull them back into outdated tendencies—including the need to be needed, and the need to serve and morph into the needs of those around them.

It may be high time to detangle what *you* want from what everyone else wants *of* you. What does living your life on your own terms even look like? Where along the way have you given up or stepped into your ethics, your desires, your power, your growth, or your integrity? Come clean and reckon with yourself to move forward.

Independent Agents and Interdependence

I have a saying I use around our house with people and pets: "We are all independent agents." It's kind of a joke because my awareness is centered in interconnectivity and interdependence, yet this perspective is helpful in living with a seven-year-old. It's also helpful for women whose awareness can get sucked into caring for others at the expense of their own health.

The pets have their own agenda (mostly napping). The kid has her own agenda. My husband and I each have our own agendas. We live together and support one another, but we take responsibility for our experience as we act in the world. The kid is being taught how to make choices to get her needs and wants met, and to be responsible for those choices. In our household, we are all life-learners—we mess up and make amends with each other. No one is in charge of making sure everyone else is happy or that the household runs smoothly. It's up to each of us how we show up and contribute as independent agents living interdependently. This is the phase we're in now—and it's taken some conscious reflection, challenging conversation, and trying on new behaviors to arrive here.

We're each responsible for how we nourish our own bodies, for how we handle situations that are not working for us, and for designing our lives in harmony together. Of course, we help and steer the seven-year-old, but the core of the lesson is that each of us largely designs our own reality, including our own physical, mental, emotional, and relational experience.

Many of my clients on this path of body thrive and spiritual evolution find, at some point, that they are surrounded by dysfunction. They realize, too, that they've played a starring role in creating or maintaining the dysfunction as the status quo of their social scene. Now they feel an uncomfortable friction. Their growth path seems to have its own agenda, while their core people seem complacently stuck.

Befriending the Unknown

One of the biggest self-sabotages in this situation is trying to figure out how it will all work out. This skips a step—a required step—which is to let go into the unknown, into the mystery, and live into the practices and habits that ignite us.

Many of us have little experience spending time in the unknown. We haven't been trained to surrender. We don't know that the unknown has its own timeline, its own intelligence. We may not trust that consciousness itself emerges when we embed the 10 Habits of Body Thrive with curiosity. Only as we walk the path with eyes wide open, in surrender to the mystery of our evolution unfolding, can we access deep wisdom.

Whoa.

I know. This is big. If you skip the unknown and try to figure out how it will all work out as you shift your relationships into alignment with who you want to become, you'll get stuck. It's impossible to figure it out from your conditioned mind. As Albert Einstein may or may not have said, "You can't solve a problem with the same thinking that created it."

Think Like Einstein

Here is a little comic relief so that you don't check out here. Albert Einstein is our familial folk hero. My dad's only memorable home decor contribution was a life-size poster of the physics genius. He pinned Albert to the wall at the bottom of the basement stairs. When I'd turn on the light to fetch something from the deep-freeze for Mom or to play a round of ping-pong with my buddies, Albert would be hanging there with his curious smile, an invitation into truth and the unknown.

Einstein wrote in a letter, "So many people today—and even professional scientists—seem to me like somebody who has seen thousands of trees but has never seen a forest." He later writes, "This independence created by philosophical insight is—in my opinion—the mark of distinction between a mere artisan or specialist and a real seeker after truth."[1]

As you navigate your higher truth via health evolution, you may indeed need to both surrender and zoom out to a bigger whole vision. Keep at the habits and push the boundaries of your own perception to access better thinking. In the process, you may awaken to relationships that need to shift or die. You won't be the only one to deal with relationship trauma, and there is comfort in knowing that this is the nature of our dynamic social evolution.

You are an independent agent, no matter how codependent your past relationships have been. You are stepping into integrity in honoring the needs of your body, mind, and spirit—meeting those needs with better daily habits. You are becoming established in yourself, what the vaidyas call *svastha*. You are becoming seated in yourself, with eyes wide open, with no strings attached, interested in growth, in connectivity, in repairing any damage done, in living ethically within yourself and betwixt your relationships. You can choose to accept the support of the unknown, of the ground of being.

You can choose to reinforce what you are stepping into in yourself with those at the frequency you want through your daily habits, friends, books, teachers, online courses, and coaches. You can intentionally cultivate a social scene that reinforces the good. And you can spend more time with yourself, with the unknown, and with the grace that arises from the ground of being, by any name.

To conclude this section, let's turn to a quote by Ayurvedic doctor Vasant Lad: "Relationships are mirrors to use for self-learning, enquiry, and investigation. Through that very learning, radical transformation of one's life can take place. If our relationships are unclear, confusion and conflict will affect our well-being."[2]

TIPS FOR NAVIGATING YOUR CORE RELATIONSHIPS AROUND HABIT CHANGE

- Return to your "why" every day. Your "why" only needs to make sense to you and will help you be centered and grounded.

- Look for support in all the right places. Don't kid yourself. Find a mentor and peers who have the habits and lifestyle you want. Join a live Body Thrive Coaching group.

- Don't sacrifice your habits for other people. You are in a tender time of transition. If you aren't true to yourself and you slide back to keep your familiar relationships stable, your integrity with yourself will diminish. Lose integrity with yourself repeatedly over time and you'll end up living someone else's life.

- With true neutrality, invite your core peeps to try what you're trying. Offer a taste or a glass of the green smoothie. Put on dance music to get the kids up in the morning before school. Never cajole, just offer.

- Schedule five-minute check-ins.

- Schedule relationship agreement conversations.

- Schedule a weekly family meeting and invite everyone to express their goals and desires. Find out how you can support each other.

- Have frank conversations. If you're curious about how your relationships could change, you need to honor your curiosity and have the conversation, even if it scares you. When you are not attached to the outcomes of your relationships, new worlds open either within the relationship, within yourself, or both.

HABIT 6

Self-Massage Your Body

WHAT TO DO

Dry-brush or oil-massage your body each day.

WHY YOU WANT TO DO IT

Your hands are your body's ultimate healing tool. The practice of daily self-massage tones your tissues, improves your sleep, stimulates your lymph, promotes longevity, strengthens your immune system, improves your joint mobility, and even synthesizes self-esteem from the inside out, which amplifies your confidence.

HOW TO START

Start with just your hands or a dry brush. Before you get dressed, simply rub your hands or a dry brush over your skin to stimulate circulation and allow your body to feel your attention and care. Eventually, graduate to giving yourself a daily oil massage to get the full benefits of self-massage.

It's early. Before the dawn. Black sky with stars. I use my hands and vigorously rub my skin awake. I use my hands and sculpt to reveal the divine within. Using circular motions around my ankles, my knees, I rouse my body with my hands for the day ahead—with my nails I scrub my scalp. With oily little fingers in my ears, I make vigorous circles. I trace around my eyes. I lift my skin from chin to temple to uplift my day. I breathe life into my cells. As I massage, I feel. As I massage, I remember. My body wasn't always this way. Years ago, some parts felt distant, disconnected. There used to be a subtle self-loathing—I'm embarrassed, yet also not embarrassed, to report—a culturally ingrained self-loathing that my body should be different than it is. This I have rubbed away over the years to heal and excavate myself. The practice takes less than five minutes.

When I rub my skin, I nourish my soul. When I don't feed my skin with self-massage, I live a less connected life. I feel less complete and start looking outside of myself for my basic bodily needs. In the practice of self-massage, you become connected to yourself as creator. As creator, you shape your body with your own hands.

Rubbing, sculpting, breathing, becoming a living soul—this is the daily practice of self-massage. In yoga philosophy, the left hand is the divine feminine; the right hand is the divine masculine. Together, you rub with the masculine and feminine forces of the divine to remember your divine nature, to connect with the paradox of duality in unity, to become powerfully alive.

This very simple practice of using your hands awakens the power in your hands to sculpt your reality. This ancient practice is called *abhyanga*. The practice of rubbing your own flesh inculcates a plethora of benefits you don't want to deny yourself, including dynamic longevity. Beauty isn't skin deep; neither is self-massage. How self-massage shapes you:

- You learn to use your own hands to help your body. As you build trust and skill over time, you become the best caretaker and healer of your body. You take your health and healing into your own hands. Your sense of touch improves, and your touch becomes a boon to others.

- You shape-shift. This practice, like the practice of yoga, opens subtle and physical channels for energy to flow. As blockages release, you shape-shift into your natural, integrated essential self.

- You become more stable, grounded, and self-contained. Getting in touch with the exterior boundaries of your body—the encasement of you—makes you less likely to be clumsy and to bump into things.

- Confidence is built from within. You'll know yourself better and discover the next level of "at-one-ment" in your own skin.

- You build your immune system. As you nourish your skin, your lymphatic system—your body's largest organ, which carries a massive load of your immune function—becomes more functional. Dry or dis-eased skin is a sign of an immune system with its guard down and gates open for germs and pathogens. If your skin is rough and dry, your plasma, the watery part of your blood, is carrying those qualities into your skin. If your skin is oily and blemished, same deal, different qualities. Nourished, attended-to skin is a protective force field.

These evolutions from self-massage happen slowly and intuitively over time, but they are the guaranteed end results of daily self-massage. An ancient *Charaka Samhita Sutrasthana* text states, "The body of one who uses oil massage regularly does not become affected much, even if subjected to accidental injuries or strenuous work. By using oil massage daily, a person is endowed with pleasant touch, trimmed body parts, and becomes strong, charming, and least affected by old age."[1]

You can tell right away when you're with someone who is comfortable in their own skin. They are relaxed, at home, at ease within themselves. There is a magnetic pull to be around them. We may sense that the tension created by our subtle self-disconnect builds walls between us. This practice enables all of us—from those who spend more time in mind than body to those with the deepest or most subtle self-loathing—to dissolve those walls.

Feed Your Skin

I mostly feed my skin with touch, fresh water, and a small amount of oil with an essential oil. Even more important than substances, I feed my skin touch. I do daily dry-brushing and a very brief daily oil massage. When you make a habit of this basic skin-nourishment routine, you check in with your limbs, joints, digits, gut, trunk, and head while feeding your skin and soul.

You need to experiment to find out which oils your skin likes best. Start with something neutral, like almond oil or sunflower oil. Sesame oil is thick and warming. Coconut oil and avocado oil are cooling. Almond and sunflower oils are in the middle. Buy cold-pressed oils in the oil section of the natural foods store. Lotion isn't the tool for the job.

What's in Your Lotion?

Oil goes rancid when exposed to water, sunlight, or air. For lotions sold commercially, chemical preservatives keep the oil from turning rancid. To boot, oil and water separate. Lotion needs emulsifiers to keep the oil and water from separating. The binding chemicals are called emulsifiers. Thus,

Lotion ≠ oil + water

Lotion = oil + water + emulsifiers + preservatives

These emulsifiers and other crap added to the oil and water destroy the sacred ecosystem of your skin, similar to how antibiotics destroy the delicate ecosystem of your gut lining and how fertilizers and pesticides contaminate our soil and waterways. As an example, here's Nivea's Pure and Natural Body Lotion ingredients list:

Water, Glycerin, Alcohol Denatured, Cetearyl
Alcohol, Isopropyl Palmitate, Glyceryl Stearate Citrate,
Octyldodecanol, Argania Spinosa Kernel Oil, Glyceryl
Glucoside, Sodium Carbomer, Methylisothiazolinone,
Phenoxyethanol, Linalool, Limonene, Citronellol, Benzyl
Alcohol, Butylphenyl Methylpropional, Alpha-Isomethyl
Ionone, Geraniol, Perfume.

Pure and natural, Nivea? My caboose. Can you feel your skin cells and blood cells screaming for protection from this complex, chemical warfare? Some ingredients in there are banned in Europe as possible human immune-system toxicants or allergens according to the Environmental Working Group.[2]

What you put on your skin, a major organ, is processed and digested by the cells. Due to toxicity, lotion stresses out your skin cells. Over time, stressed-out cells malfunction. The chemicals go through your skin into your bloodstream and get captured by your liver. If you use lotion, look up the chemicals. Decide if you want those chemicals in your liver.

Experiment to notice the difference between using lotion and oil. Lotion keeps your awareness at skin level. Oil opens the connection between you and your deeper bodily tissues—your muscles, bones, blood, nerves. Where there is connection, consciousness flows, and intelligence moves and informs. When you use lotion, you miss out on plugging your cells into the intelligence that formed you.

Each morning after I shower, I lightly towel off, keeping some moisture on my skin. If I'm in a warm climate, I rub some coconut oil between my hands. If I'm in a cold climate, I use sesame oil. I give my body a nice five-minute massage, hitting everywhere I can reach, which is everywhere.

First, I rub up and down my long bones and circle my joints. Parts of my body call for attention—my lost horizons of stagnation: hips, thighs, booty. When I'm not looking, emotions and cellulite glue themselves to those big muscles. It pays off big for me to spend a few extra moments loving my legs, dissolving stagnation with my hands.

The practice of self-massage is lavishly healing. Time changes the body. You can intentionally embrace the changes of time and insert daily sacred practices that protect, heal, preserve, and enlighten. When you devote yourself to self-improvement and long-term health, this practice is indispensable.

Read the instructions below and ask yourself "What is *doable* for me right now?" and "What do I *want* to do?"

Quick Instructions: Without Oil

If you've never done self-massage and you're tweaked out about an oily mess, then start with dry-hand massage. Give yourself a good, thorough shakedown with your hands in the morning before getting dressed. Start with one limb at a time. Long strokes on the long bones. Round strokes at the joints. Listen to what your body wants.

If you'd like to stimulate and exfoliate your skin, buy a dry brush or exfoliating gloves at a natural foods store in the self-care section. Lightly scrub yourself awake, avoiding sensitive areas. Dry-brushing is simple, fast, not messy, and fantastic for circulation.

Quick Instructions: With Oil

Oil adds another dimension to the daily ritual. Pure oil is pure fat. Inside your body the function of fat tissue is to lubricate the physical and emotional body. The Sanskrit word *sneha* translates as both "oil" and "love." High-functioning fat tissue engenders emotional ease through our facility to love and be loved. We become relaxed and available for deep connectedness. When fat tissue is deficient, disconnect occurs from the field and availability of love, as intrinsically arising and available through relationships: relationship with cosmos, with self, with community. When fat tissue is excessive, it becomes dense, white fat. Excess white fat indicates not only diseases of stagnation, but also from an Ayurvedic perspective an emotional clinginess or attachment. Unprocessed physical toxins and unprocessed emotional hurts hide in excess white fat tissue.

What does this have to do with rubbing oil on your body? The practice of self-massage with oil, or abhyanga, is hands-on connectivity with you and your fat tissue. If you have mounds on your belly, thighs, or chest, the friction of the massage, done in a loving way, stimulates the processing of excess fat tissue, and paradoxically helps build deficient fat tissue. If your fat tissue is already healthy, you open the door for taking your hands-on healing skills and body integrity to the next level through upping the ante on the intimacy of self-care.

You can give yourself a quick massage just based on a physical practice. Yet the practice itself, when done consistently over time, will engender a deeper level of self-love. Any subtle self-discontent or self-loathing, whether it's at the physical or mental-emotional level, eventually gives way to higher, more integrated emotional connectivity. Here are the steps for oil massage:

1. Use the oil that is best for your body type. (Take an online dosha quiz: bodythrive.com/quiz.) If you are:
   - vata predominant, use untoasted sesame oil.
   - pitta predominant, use coconut oil in summer, sunflower oil in winter.
   - kapha predominant, use a mix of corn and untoasted sesame oil.

2. Put your oil in a four-ounce massage-oil bottle or old, sterilized mustard bottle.

3. Warm it before use by placing the bottle in a coffee cup filled with hot water.

4. Massage enough oil into your skin to feel lubricated, but not greasy. The amount depends on your body type and climate. (Dry people in a desert need more oil than oily people in the tropics!) Start with one limb at a time. Use long strokes on the long bones and round strokes at the joints. Listen to what your body wants. Massage all parts: limbs, hands, feet, belly, chest, neck, head. Move from your head toward your toes for relaxing, from your toes toward your head for stimulating, or push everything to the digestive tract for detoxing.

5. Shower to rinse off the extra oil.

6. Use an old towel to pat yourself dry.

Extra-Quick Instructions   Keep your oil in the shower. After you're warm, turn off the shower. Spend a moment massaging the oil into your skin. Give yourself a quick rinse, and pat dry.

Once-a-Week Long-Massage Instructions   Find a nice, sunny, indoor spot and give yourself a longer massage. Play relaxing music. Make a cup of tea. Get out an old towel and sit on the floor. Take time to sculpt yourself and breathe life into your flesh and soul. Work the oil deep into your skin. Enjoy. Sit in silence. Then, rinse off.

Tales of Self-Massage

This sacred daily habit, above all the others, has the strongest effect on creating bodily self-love. Here are stories about self-massage from members of the online Body Thrive group:

> **Cindy**   "I am now consistently doing oil self-massage. I am more juicy, lustrous, calm. My pains are nourished into juicy (hip, knee) joints. My stress is decreased. I can't help but feel this has certainly strengthened my immune function. Oil massage lets me 'pause' and reframe my tendency to be irritable. I feel my cells rest into comfort as I seal in love."

> **Charis**   "Oil massage has been amazing. I've been doing it at night as part of my bedtime routine before I take a shower, and I sleep so much better. My skin isn't itchy and is less cracked from the dry desert weather. I've been able to wake up before my alarm! I love, love, love this practice."

> **Dana**   "I do my sesame-oil massage in the morning. After yoga, before showering. Inspired, I changed the bedtime routine of my kids. They don't get to watch a short film before bed anymore. We

started clearing the apartment of kids' clutter (new habit) after brushing the teeth (trigger), and the reward is a foot massage or some other part that they demand. We all love the new routine!"

Shinay "I do it every day. I feel more grounded, more loved (by my own self), and much more nourished. I also find that I need to eat less oil and fats in general the more oil I put on my skin."

Amy "At first, abhyanga was more of a 'to do' thing to check off as one of my new, daily self-care practices. Now, I try to bring in more of an emotional quality to it, even if I am just doing a quick morning rubdown. I appreciate my body and send it loving-kindness. I feel like I notice what's going on through my skin and tissue. It gives me a sense of protection. This practice builds appreciation and care for myself over time."

SELF-MASSAGE FAQS

Can I just use a dry brush?

If you have dry skin, don't just use a dry brush—it's stimulating and drying. If you have dry skin, but you are using lotion, stop that and start using oil. If you don't have dry skin, dry-brushing is invigorating and can be done daily. However, try oil massage now and then to experience the emotional connection that oil facilitates.

Do I get the same benefits from my foam roller?

Foam-rolling relaxes your muscles and stimulates your lymph, similar to self-massage. The differences are that you don't get the benefits of the oil lubrication, and you don't use your hands on your body. There is a deeper emotional-body connection with oil massage. All that said, foam-rolling is the bomb and falls somewhere between this practice and the breath-body practices.

I can't stand the intimacy of self-massage. Do I have to do this practice?

Start with a dry brush. The barrier between your hands and skin will help you get started. This practice will slowly dissolve the rift between your desire for wellness and your ability to self-nurture. After a spell, instead of the brush, you may be ready to use your hands and oil.

Can I do this after my shower instead of before?

Sure. I have old plumbing and find that after the shower works better for me. Use oil sparingly on damp skin, and use an old towel to remove excess oil so your clothes don't become oily.

Do you have a tip sheet on self-massage?

Yes, Dos and Don'ts for Self-Massage can be found in the online *Body Thrive Workbook*. Print it and put it in your bathroom until this habit becomes an automated part of your daily routine.

Does massage from my partner or massage therapist count?

Receiving massage from others is lovely; however, unless you can afford to hire someone, other people will quickly lose interest in giving you a daily massage. The benefit of this particular practice is to train your own hands to safeguard your own flesh.

How long should I massage my baby and young kids?

You can massage your kids for as long as they will let you. Prioritize frequency over length. Two to ten minutes is plenty of time to rub enough oil into their skin, strengthen their immune function, help them relax, and train them to receive healing touch.

Can my kids do their own massage?

Self-massage and dry brushing are normal human behavior around my house. Since my daughter was born, I've followed her bath with a five-minute oil massage routine that gives me a chance to check in with her body. Though she is now old enough to massage herself, she would still rather relax and receive. I have no doubt that her exceptionally loving and affectionate personality was nurtured by our massage habit. And I have no doubt that in a year or so, she'll do the practice by herself. Steer toward autonomy.

If I do this before I shower, will there be oil stuck in my drain?

This is a probability. The more oil you use, the more will go down the drain. If you have old plumbing, use oil sparingly, clean your drains frequently, or do oil massage *after* your shower or bath. Once a week, clean your drains with a small amount of ecofriendly drain cleanser.

My towels and clothes are oily. Am I doing something wrong?

You are using more oil than your skin can absorb. Use less oil, or mix a little oil with water to thin it out in your hands before you rub it into your skin. Dry off with old towels. Put your towels through the wash with a heavy-duty mechanics' detergent, like Permatex.

My shower/tub is slippery from the oil. Help!

If you're worried about slipping, use oil *after* you shower. Or keep a big sponge and a bottle of dish detergent in your shower. At the end of your shower, wash the shower with your feet and the sponge. If you share a shower, make sure the floor is free from oil so you don't take out the next user.

Should I incorporate acupressure and essential oils?

Self-massage opens the doorway for you to explore your body with your hands. Both Ayurveda and Chinese medicine detail an array of *marma* points and acupressure points that stimulate your biochemistry. You can make your own body oils to balance your doshas and chakras. There is so much to learn when it comes to awakening your hands to heal, yet the magnificent message is simply to start and to commit to the habit as a practice of self-care.

What is the kaizen approach to starting self-massage?

1. Use an anchor statement like "I appreciate my body" or "I use my hands to heal."

2. Start with one-minute dry-brushing or self-massage without oil. Hold yourself back. Do this every morning before getting dressed.

3. After a few weeks, increase your massage to two to five minutes.

4. After a few months, start giving yourself an oil massage before or after you shower.

5. After a few more months, add a longer session once a week to once a month.

HABIT 7

Sit in Silence

WHAT TO DO

Take some time each day, preferably at the same time, to sit in silence. Simply stop, drop, and sit.

WHY YOU WANT TO DO IT

To live empowered, you need to clear your mind and digest your experiences. Sitting purposefully in silence, you digest your thoughts, ideas, and experiences. You become available to profound insights and bigger perspectives. You gain access to inner freedom. You tap into a big-time, big-space perspective, which erases the effects of earthly stress. You learn how to learn and how to align directly from consciousness, from source. You subtly allow the fabric of your physiology to knit together in a subtle vibratory field, which lends itself to higher immune integration and tissue rejuvenation.

HOW TO START

Set an alert on your smartphone to stop, drop, and sit. Then use the timer on your phone. Start with a

one-minute practice. Sit with an erect spine on the edge
of your chair or on a cushion. Choose to open or close
your eyes. Relax. Allow your awareness to expand. Relax.
Be aware. Make room for everything to be as it is, without needing to change anything. Stop; time is up.

When I first realized that someone, somewhere in the world was
already meditating whenever I sat to practice, something shifted for
me. Someone—hopefully hundreds of thousands of someones—at
that very moment, on this very planet, was already co-creating a strong
meditative field. All I had to do was join them in the etheric realm, in
the space between us.

Information Overload Has Implications

We have more data to consume than time or gray matter. If you tip the
scales toward overstimulation with too many calls, texts, emails, pod-
casts, videos, or screens, you destroy the very channels in your subtle
nervous system physiology in which the information and energy are
moving. Through excess stimulation and overuse, you wear out the
container that holds prana, energy, and ideas. You are wired and tired.

In modern society, information overload is taking its toll. We're
all affected. If you choose *not* to unplug and unwind, you implode.
Although it may seem like a personal struggle—a personal issue—it's
not. It's epidemic and impersonal. The dis-eases of the digital age
erode your peace of mind and your immune function, or ojas.

If you keep this up for long, you render yourself exhausted, having
eroded your nerves, the containers that carry life force. In Ayurveda,
that container is likened to a bucket that holds life force. Overstimulation causes holes and cracks in the bucket—energy leaks out instead of
being put to good use. You frazzle and disintegrate your nerves.

Every byte of information or stimulation you consume through
your senses, consciously or unconsciously, must be digested. Digestion

requires space, time, and the fire of awareness. Similar to how over-eating taxes your digestive fire and renders you subpar, overexposure to mental and sensory data taxes your mental agni, rendering your decision-making apparatus subpar.

The intensity you live in needs an equal and opposite spaciousness to decompress. This is the law of pulsation, called *spanda*. Otherwise, burnout becomes inevitable. Autoimmune issues, sleep issues, endocrine issues, nervous-system issues, and even asthma (which can be linked to anxiety) slowly take up residence and are formidable to evict. On the digital battlefield, your temporal opponents are information overload and hyperconnectivity.

Meditation Is Our Secret Weapon, Our Savior, and Our Salve

You are wired to connect, to interconnect, to act, and to create. Inversely, you are also wired to simply be, to be silent, and to experience pure receptivity and effortlessness. As a culture, we are running a deficit in the latter, the stress of which is creating a slew of imbalances.

Balance is a pulsation of the opposites moving on an evolutionary trajectory. It is a slide on a spectrum of opposites, a moving target relying on the law of pulsation. The opposites pulsate: empty/full, stillness/movement, hunger/satiation, hot/cold, heavy/light. The opposite of action is the deliberate inaction of meditation. And yet, *being* is a verb with an opposite action of *doing*. Non-doing is the doing of being, which makes it challenging to learn.

Sitting in silence, or meditation, is a core human competency that teaches us, on increasingly subtle levels, acceptance, patience, ease, trust, and how to let go into source, into the universe that created us. Sitting in silence, you let go to free yourself from the whims of the mind, to receive and be nourished, all from the place of not doing. You access being as the backdrop to doing.

That shift has more than a few benefits. To illuminate why you want to meditate, let's go to the end of the first book in the Yoga Sutras of Patanjali, the ancient yoga bible:

As one gains proficiency in the undisturbed flow of consciousness that occurs beyond subtle thought, a purity and luminosity of the inner instrument of mind is developed.

(nirvichara vaisharadye adhyatma prasadah)

The experiential knowledge that is gained in that state is one of essential wisdom and is filled with truth.

(ritambhara tatra prajna)

That knowledge is different from the knowledge that is commingled with testimony or through inference, because it relates directly to the specifics of the object, rather than to those words or other concepts.

(shruta anumana prajnabhyam anya-vishaya vishesha-arthatvat)

This type of knowledge that is filled with truth creates latent impressions in the mind-field, and those new impressions tend to reduce the formation of other less useful forms of habitual latent impressions.

(tajjah samskarah anya samskara paribandhi)[1]

These sutras are saying that meditation enables your mind to rewire itself straight from consciousness, changing the way your brain works. The big problem in upgrading habits is that your past habits have both a mind (mental pattern) of their own and a momentum—or *samskara*, as indicated in the last sutra.

If you are the sum of your habits and experiences, then to grow, you need to reprogram your habits and experiences. Upgrading the impressions in your mind-field undermines the momentum of your outdated habits. By meditating, you're upgrading the hardwiring of your operating system with access to a greater truth, or smarter impressions, and a more connected view of reality.

How Meditation Works

From brain science, we know that stress shuts down the frontal lobe, thus disabling higher-order thinking. The primitive brain, or brain stem, is active when you're stressed, turning on your impulsive, reactive, fearful, and addicted tendencies. When you meditate, the blood flow to your brain moves from the primitive brain to the prefrontal cortex, or the front of the frontal lobe.[2] This movement shifts you from being reactive to receptive, from impulsive and anxious to clear and kind, from compulsive to creative.

Meditation builds brain cells, increases gray matter, and allows the brain to slow responses to stress, providing better concentration, learning, and memory.[3] This simple practice thickens the part of your brain that makes decisions while shrinking the part of your brain that is active during the fight-or-flight response. Personally, I'd rather make better decisions than be stuck in a postmodern fight-or-flee response.

In Ayurveda, this is recognized as a shift from operating from the lower egoic mind, named *ahamkara*, to the higher, spiritually awake mind, called *buddhi*. Meditation activates buddhi, which is the conscious choice-maker that supersedes the subconscious mind. With choice comes empowerment. By taking time to meditate, you can digest your past emotions, thoughts, and experiences so they don't hijack your future.

Getting Over the Overwhelm

Today, the "I-me-my" perspective dominates. Personal busyness and overwhelm is the modern default way of orienting. On an epidemic scale, overwhelm leads you to be less aware of the needs of yourself, others, and the planet. The stakes are high to transform overwhelm to openness.

Even for those who aren't overloaded, overscheduled, overthinking, or over "it," you still have a core human need to meditate. If you are, indeed, on a strong self-evolution path, meditation weakens the ties to your outdated, stale, and pathological mental and emotional patterning. Neural plasticity increases as you rewire your brain into your wide-open potential. As your meditation practice develops, your outdated patterns become clear. Time and space open up. You make new, intentionally designed choices and assume a more evolved identity. Thus, you're taking charge to disengage the number-one cause of disease: making careless choices. Plus, like all of the 10 Habits of Body Thrive, meditation is free!

Do You Have Time *Not* to Meditate?

Many of my clients and students tell me they don't have time to meditate. I understand. I still go through phases of my life when I almost convince myself that I don't have time to meditate. At times, I even believe myself for two consecutive weeks despite more than fifteen years of practice that prove contrary to this notion. Inevitably, I experience (a) stress, (b) inefficient use of time, (c) poor sleeping habits, (d) gross-level thinking, and (e) dramatic or subtle negative emotions. I lose the platform of living my day from a bigger perspective. I lose access to deep space, deep time, and subtle awareness. I become ordinary and stuck in the "I-me-my" mindset, which defaults toward the narcissistic, materialistic, self-righteous, and petty. In a nutshell, I become small-minded.

Once I notice, my *tejas* (light of awareness) and my *viveka* (ability to call myself out on my own hogwash) kick in—I call my own bluff, and it's back to the cushion. For those who are experienced meditators, take a moment to write down what happens when you don't meditate for a spell. Get curious. Be honest. Use that as fuel to begin practice anew.

Rebecca Gladding, MD, coauthor of *You Are Not Your Brain*, describes the benefits of sitting daily:

> Sitting every day, for at least fifteen to thirty minutes, makes a huge difference in how you approach life, how personally you take things, and how you interact with others. It enhances compassion, allows you to see things more clearly (including yourself) and creates a sense of calm and centeredness that is indescribable. There really is no substitute.[4]

Unstick Your Samskaras

If you've never had a meditation practice, you may be unaware of how you perpetuate your own mental-emotional pattern. Stuck in the pattern, you're more likely to buy into your own thoughts and limiting beliefs. For example, a belief might be, "I don't have time to meditate." You'll look for evidence to back that up and find plenty. You can also find lots of stuck company. But stuck is stagnant. When you're in a stagnant pattern, you repeat the same conversations, internally and with other people, as the scenery changes. You don't change or grow. You don't break the bounds of your self-imposed imprisonment. If you are complacent, you barricade the door to your potential.

To break the cycle, you need skin in the game of waking up. You need to pay to play. You need to overcome your excuses and your resistance. Find a teacher. Make your practice a habit. As motivational author Steven Pressfield advises, "Turn pro" with your life. Come to your mat with your game on, ready for a breakthrough. Otherwise, you'll stop, drop, and daydream. And stagnate.

In the post-information connection-conceptual economy, humans are waking up to self-awareness in droves. Great meditation teachings, which are freed of cultural dogma, have streamlined the process of letting go and waking up. Now is a wonderful time to become a meditator or to help others who want the benefits of stopping, dropping, and sitting. Learn to relax and pay attention. Don't make it any more difficult than that.

Learning Meditation: Relax and Pay Attention

Because meditation is difficult to learn from reading a book, find an audio practice either online or on an app. You'll find it easier to be guided when it's time to meditate.

The best basic instruction is to "relax and pay attention." Pay attention to what, you ask? Pay attention to your power of attention. Attend to attention itself. Relax while attending to momentary presence. Let go, be aware. As you let go, your awareness shifts inward. Presence has a levity and a gravity. Allow yourself to be pulled into the natural gravity of deep presence, wholeness, and fulfillment. Try it for one minute now. I'll pause and join you.

How did it go? Are you a smidgen more relaxed, at ease, or tuned in to your bodily needs? Meditation gravitates us toward spiritual fulfillment, mental clarity, emotional release, bodily health, and interpersonal connectivity.

If you experienced the opposite—more stress or more anxiety—be gentle with yourself. You need to learn the process of relaxation.

You can work yourself into a tizzy noticing a flood of thoughts, memories, or projections. If meditation makes you anxious, return again and again to the "relax" instruction. Allow your breath to breathe you. You may find a gateway in lying down and feeling the earth support your body. That is a more relaxing way to start.

During meditation, you make consistent micro-choices on increasingly subtle realms while in a deeply relaxed state and safe space. This is how the decision-making part of your brain grows while the impulsive part of your brain shrinks. The choices you are making while you are meditating go something like this: Should I scratch that itch? Can I relax more? Should I stop daydreaming? Should I stop early to send that email?

At first, you start to see your thoughts, emotions, and feelings from a distance. The more you return to the practice and let the riff do its thing without shifting your attention to it, the more your brain chemistry smartens up.

By making the choice to relax and pay attention, again and again, moment by moment, you generate friction, similar to rubbing the genie out of the lamp. The result? You release your inner genie, who grants you expanded consciousness, upgraded awareness, more brain cells, more sensitivity, and more creativity. And, while you meditate, your body experiences deep rest and tissue repair. The hitch? It only lasts a day. Then, you need to rub your genie out of the bottle again.

The Paradox of Meditation

Meditation is paradoxical. If you get stressed from meditating, this means you naturally spend more time in "alert" mode than in "relaxed" mode. You need to learn "relax." For those who fall asleep, either you need to return to Habit 2, Go to Bed Early, or you need to learn how to wake up and pay attention.

Whatever your tendency, with practice, that tendency—and even the paradox—dissolves. Meditation is a verb, not a noun. It has the rub of the opposites of relaxing and paying attention brushing against each other, creating the friction of your evolution. To become whole, you dance the paradox until it dissolves into unity. Time meets timelessness; the parts amalgamate into the whole.

The Paradox of Meditation	
Relax	Pay attention
Release	Be alert
Let go	Sit upright
Be restful	Become awake

Between relaxing and attending, you let go of the world, of busyness, and dissolve into higher mind. You melt into the wholeness of your deep, unlimited presence.

The increasingly subtle action of meditation is paying attention to your power of attention. When you wander into thinking, recollecting, or planning, stop. Relax and pay attention to attention itself. When you're quiet enough, you can feel your brain chemistry interconnecting.

Am I Doing It Right?

"Am I doing it right?" This is the most common question from beginners and experienced meditators alike. One way to know is how you feel after, not during, your practice. Signs that your practice is working:

- You don't feel as rushed. You may feel calm and at ease.

- You notice more detail, including the sky and the trees.

- You experience more gratitude and less fear.

- Your perspective is widening.

- Your field of compassion expands and empathy deepens.

- Your attention is less self-absorbed.

- You are becoming more open minded.

- You listen deeply.

- You experience clarity.

- You are happier, positive, and uplifted.

- You enjoy your life and celebrate others.

- When you feel stressed or out of balance, you stop, drop and sit.

What Happens to Meditators

Ask any seasoned meditator about the benefits they've experienced through meditation and watch what happens in their eyes. Watch their eyes brighten and dilate. To meditate is to dive into the realm of our expanding universe firsthand. Our insides open up. When I asked my teacher Craig Hamilton what meditation has taught him, he said, "I've learned to free-fall backward, unknowing and without fear, through my day-to-day life."

The deep letting go of meditation translates into everyday awareness by enabling you to be present without projection and without preference. You avail yourself of both the presence of being and the possibility of becoming.

You get around and beyond yourself. "To know the self, we must go beyond the mind" is a common Eastern mystical teaching. After your practice, you can see your thoughts and emotions for what they are. You can plug in or let go, intentionally engaging that which you want to think and create. You can easily drop or disengage from outdated thoughts or beliefs and old emotional patterns.

For me, the deep letting go, the backward free-fall is a deep *diksha*, or rite of passage, of meditation and living awake. For advanced meditators, the effort—or *tapas*—of the practice becomes increasingly subtle. Patterns emerge at every plateau.

Next-level breakthroughs eventually require a bigger "why" and the power of a posse exploring the new frontier of collective awakening. If this grabs your attention, check out a meditation community with Patricia Albere, Jeff Carreira, or Craig Hamilton.

Build Your Meditation Ritual

You know how to adopt a new habit; you know that the preconditions for progress are (1) you have to want to do it, and (2) you have to perceive it as doable.

The name of the game is making a meditation habit into a ritual. Rituals are practiced, sequential actions that conserve and streamline decision-making energy. Authors Jim Loehr and Tony Schwartz discuss this idea in their book *The Power of Full Engagement*: "We use the word 'ritual' purposefully to emphasize the notion of a carefully defined, highly structured behavior. In contrast to will and discipline, which require pushing yourself to a particular behavior, a ritual pulls at you. The power of rituals is that they insure that we use as little conscious energy as possible where it is not absolutely necessary, leaving us free to strategically focus the energy available to us in creative, enriching ways."[5]

Loehr and Schwartz underline that managing energy, not time, is the key to high performance and personal renewal. In this current heyday of complexity, information overload, and decision fatigue, you want to make a decision once and commit. Like habit guru James Clear lays out in his blog post, "How Willpower Works: The Science of Decision Fatigue and How to Avoid Bad Decisions," you want to:

- plan daily decisions before it's time to take action.
- do the most important thing first.
- stop making decisions and start making commitments.[6]

Decide if you're going to be a meditator right now in this life-cycle phase or not. If not, that's okay; revisit this chapter later. If so, proceed with making the when, where, and how decision. In Loehr and Schwartz lingo, "Emphasize the notion of a carefully defined, highly structured behavior," then commit to those behaviors.[7]

For meditation, break down the activity like a Catholic priest preparing and delivering Mass. This is the time of day. This is what you wear. This is how long you sit. This is what you sit on. This is how you sit. You may even state your intention aloud. Then you begin. You practice. The buzzer goes off. You're done. You bow. You fold your clothes. The ritual is over. Set this up and make these choices before it's time to meditate.

Make these decisions ahead of time by architecting your environment and rehearsing the ritual. If meditation is more important to you right now than breath-body practices, then do it first. Commit so you don't need to entertain the if, when, where, or how you should meditate every day. Plan ahead and make fewer decisions in your day. Set up your outer environment to encourage the budding habit.

Again, paraphrasing William Durant's ideas: "Excellence is an art won by training and habituation."[8] To become an excellent, effective meditator, break down the steps to getting to your seat and shifting your awareness into a more subtle knowing. Don't waste energy deciding each day *if* you are going to meditate.

Loehr and Schwartz emphasize, "All great performers rely on positive rituals to manage their energy and regulate their behavior."[9] Simply decide for this phase of your life if it's worth a few minutes of your day, and if it is, you have to decide to commit. Then, make it doable.

Let's investigate the relationship between good habits and rituals. Both are commitments usually initiated with a purpose and an intention and worked toward automation. Yet, a deeper meaning and a level of complexity both upgrade a habit into a ritual. Good habits, like brushing and flossing, don't require a deeper meaning as rituals do.

Meditation can be more easily automated and enhanced by ritual. Though you can make a habit of sitting daily for fifteen minutes, you'll gain more traction in your progress when you make your practice sacred. The heart you put into the small actions of preparing to practice, practicing, and emerging from your practice make meditation a ritual. Meaning will pull you into the ritual, thus freeing up more focus for the practice itself. For meditation to be more effective, make it sacred.

The Power of Pranayama

Before concluding the Sit in Silence habit, I want to shine a light on pranayama. For many, it's easier to "just sit" if you start with a "just sit and breathe" practice.

Ayurveda and yoga use pranayama as a cure-all rejuvenator and full body-mind elixir. Breathing occurs primarily through involuntary muscles. When you breathe consciously, you shift to voluntary control of your breath. You shift your mind from reactive to generative. Through deep conscious breathing, you can lower your heartbeat and oxygenate the lower lobes of your lungs, where your relaxation receptors reside. You can switch from a state of deoxygenated stress. Ayurvedic doc John Douillard explains it like this: "Nose breathing drives oxygen more efficiently into the lower lobes of the lungs rather than staying in the upper lobes, as with mouth breathing. With nose breathing, all five lobes of the lungs are used to breathe rather than just the upper two. The lower lobes of the lungs, have more parasympathetic, calming, and repairing nerve receptors, which are activated during nose breathing exercise. The upper lobes have more sympathetic (fight-or-flight) stress receptors that are activated during mouth breathing exercise."[10]

When you breathe with depth and fullness, you open the space around your organs, spine, and digestive tract, and you activate your parasympathetic nervous system (PNS). When your PNS is flipped on, your mood lifts and you experience *sukha* (ease) and *ananda* (good feelings or bliss). You unlock the treasure trove of your biochemistry. Expand your exhale to deepen your inhale. You build lung capacity and bliss capacity over time. Your innards become more perceivable, interconnected, conscious, and awake.

The pranayama habit compounds to grow your capacity—you expand your lungs, you absorb more life force, you experience both subtler and more powerful fields of energy. The Kripalu Center for Yoga and Health website explains it this way:

> Yoga teaches that the human nervous system has potentials
> far beyond the normal regulation of the physical and
> mental bodies. In yoga, the human nervous system is like
> a set of antennae that can focus and channel the creative

power of the universe into expression in a single life. Pranayama practice polishes the capacity of the nervous system to conduct this cosmic creative potential into real, tangible manifestation. It is similar to increasing the capacity of the wires and filament inside a light bulb so that it can handle more wattage without burning out. When the wires can handle more wattage, it produces more light and heat. When we practice deep breathing every day, our subtle wiring gradually becomes stronger, and we begin to fill up with light and energy. In many ways, this is all we really mean when we talk about being "enlightened." There is really no end point, just a gradually increasing capability of our nervous system to handle all forms of energy.[11]

When you do conscious breath-body work daily (and pranayama is considered a breath-body practice), you experience more spaciousness and freedom inside yourself—more room to move, more peace in your emotions and relations. When you slow the breath, you slow your perception of time. You will experience deep time and deep space. When you notice the pause between the breaths, you notice that life has pauses—it's not always full bore ahead.

After you take time to breathe in the morning, you will be aware during the day of pauses between activities, choice points in your mental and emotional patterns, and choice points in your words and behaviors. It becomes easier to shift into who you want to be and how you want to show up for your life, including how you want to show up for everyone else.

With pranayama, you become more sensitive and aware of others' needs and potential, and of the collaborative opportunities for elevated interconnection. You can expand your breath, your perspective, and the possibilities in any moment, no matter what is happening with whom. If you take time to breathe before bed, you process the day and sleep more deeply.

Pranayama infuses your biochemistry with love, balances your hormones, decelerates every measurable marker of aging, wires a stronger energetic capacity, and enables access to inner peace. And pranayama is free, always available, requires no equipment, and painlessly lowers the barrier to entry.

TIPS FOR SITTING IN SILENCE

- If you resist meditation, start with a one-minute deep-breathing practice. Bring 100 percent of your awareness to that one-minute practice. Try one minute before sleep and one minute as part of your Start the Day Right habit.

- Sit in the same place at the same time each day. Very early morning is the best time for most people.

- Bring in ritual.

- For guided instruction, use an audio recording, if desired, or a meditation app like Headspace, which has teachings and habit tracking.

- Set the timer on your phone. When the timer goes off, stop—even if you want to keep going. Potent, regular practice is better than sporadic, longer practice.

- Gradually increase the length of practice. Don't set yourself up for failure by making your sit time too long. Work your way up, first to five minutes, then gradually to ten. Increase by five-minute increments until you're happy with your results. While thirty minutes twice a day works great for many serious meditators, remember the practice needs to work for you right now in your life. Use kaizen to make meditation an effortless daily routine, building your meditation muscle consistently.

- If you used to meditate and you've strayed, try restarting with five, ten, or fifteen minutes—whatever you can commit to *daily* during this phase of your life.

- If you started daydreaming, planning, problem-solving, worrying, remembering, or reminiscing, know that is where meditation becomes a practice. None of these mentioned actions is as basic as resting in awareness. In this practice, we're tapping into the backdrop of life. Some call it the ground of being. When you notice you're in the forefront of your normal repetitive mental patterns, gently and quickly nudge your attention back to attention itself.

- Find other meditators. Tap into what is already happening on the frequency you want to live into. Your practice will stabilize and advance. Don't go it alone.

HABIT 8

Heed the Healthier Eating Guidelines

WHAT TO DO

Eat only two or three meals a day, without snacking. You'll burn fat between meals and be hungry to thoroughly enjoy them. Reconnect with the chicken-scratching sensation in your stomach, signifying readiness to eat, and you will provoke a deeper, fat-burning metabolism. Empower your digestion to work undisturbed by taking only water between meals.

WHY YOU WANT TO DO IT

Nourishment is as much about *when* you eat and *how* you eat as it is about what you eat. When you eat only a few times a day, you burn fat, a steady energy source, between meals. This habit of honoring emptiness and fullness, rest and digestion, and hunger and satiation attunes you to the law of pulsation for maximum energy.

Digestion requires energy. When you eat emotionally, or too frequently, you tax your digestion, rendering less energy available for everything else you want to do. If you tax your digestion repeatedly, a residue of poorly digested food builds up in your gastrointestinal (GI) tract. The buildup is grime in your physical, mental, and emotional gears. Uplevel your energy and cultivate deep power by improving your digestion.

HOW TO START

Before you take a bite, take a breath. Make sure you're hungry. If you've had a meal in the last one to three hours, drink water and take a short walk instead. Chances are you're looking for a distraction or you're thirsty.

My friend Hunter, a local cabinetmaker and seasonal big-game hunter, came to see me about digestive complaints. I asked him to stick out his tongue. I wanted to see and smell what was going on in his digestive tract. The tongue and breath do not lie. Through my Ayurvedic practice, I've noticed that the client's body is often more descriptive and accurate than their words.

A thick white coating of ama covered Hunter's tongue. Under the coating, red dots were poking through. I asked Hunter if he ate leftovers. He proudly replied, "I make a crock of stew or something on Sundays and eat it for the week." Aha.

Uh-oh.

Food starts to lose prana, life-force energy, when it is left overnight, even in the fridge. Your food should taste and feel vibrant with life force. You may have noticed that flavor fades from leftovers and they require more salt to be palatable, which is more sodium for your body to process. Your tongue is your body's gatekeeper, detecting the freshness, flavor, or lack thereof. Your tongue is also the ambassador of the entire GI tract, and as such, it decides what to swallow and what to spit out.

You want your tongue to be smart, alert, and ready to inform you whether you should ingest or eject a particular food.

Your Snakelike Digestive Tract

Your digestive tract is like a snake, with its head being the tongue and tail being the anus. Your tongue also has a map of the whole snake, which you can check on the tongue illustrations in Habit 9, page 183. Your tongue, as GI ambassador, gets to choose whether to swallow or spit.

However, due to poor digestion, you may have a thick coating on your tongue that causes you to lose the sharp clarity of your taste buds. A coated tongue can't taste accurately, and it makes a horrible ambassador for the deeper tissue of the body, which depends on the tongue to meet its nutritional and taste requirements.

A healthy tongue looks vibrant, pink, and moist with a thin, almost clear coating. It tastes accurately. Your tongue, the ambassador of your digestion, communicates what the deeper tissue of your body wants. If your taste buds and guts are healthy, you'll be receptive only to healthy foods. If your deeper tissue is mixed with ama, your tongue will be receptive to addictive and nonnutritive foods. For example, if you are an adult who doesn't drink soda or eat nonnutritive chips, you're repelled by them. If you're addicted to nonnutritive foods and beverages, this addiction reflects the cellular confusion caused by those substances. As you comply with the following Healthier Eating Guidelines and nourish yourself with a plant-based diet, that cellular confusion is upgraded to cellular intelligence.

The Healthier Eating Guidelines (HEGs)

The HEGs are basic rules for attuning your tongue, listening to your gut, and nourishing yourself. They read like a rule book. You may find some of the rules too challenging for you right now. Recall your "what" and your "why" on your journey to Body Thrive (see A Crash Course on Habit Evolution, page 19).

Read the HEGs below and check off two that you want to work on. Or if you suffer from poor digestion or elimination, insomnia, or stress, find which guidelines you break the most. Make those your new habits.

- Eat only two to three times a day, when hungry (not bored, tired, thirsty, or upset).

- Take only water, without ice, between meals to let your digestion rest.

- Live on fresh food. Make your food daily. Don't live on leftovers, frozen foods, canned foods, or the prepared foods from the grocery store. Notice the prana in fresh.

- Pause in gratitude and receptivity for your food and those who contributed to its journey to your body.

- Do not eat when emotionally distracted or multitasking.

- Enjoy your food. Taste the tastes.

- Relax after eating. After a big meal, rest for five to fifteen minutes, then take a stroll if you can.

- Steer toward high-nutrient foods.

- Slow down for a satisfying midday meal.

- Eat a light dinner, leaving time to digest before rest.

- Allow thirteen hours between dinner and "breaking" your fast.

- Be like Goldilocks—find just the right amount to eat so you don't stretch your stomach *or* need to eat too frequently.

- Eat during daylight hours.

- Incorporate the six tastes explained on pages 169–171.

- Follow Ayurveda's food-combining rules explained on page 176.

- Learn the best diet for your Ayurvedic constitution and time of life.

- Eat your ecosystem. You'll eat seasonally and locally, and be more connected to stewarding your hood.

As a rule-breaker, I've broken all of these Healthier Eating Guidelines. When I first encountered Ayurveda, I was breaking most of them. Over the last seventeen years, I've tested each of the HEGs and found that, indeed, my overall health improves with each rule. The goal isn't perfection—it's great digestion. Stop obstructing your body from receiving nutrition, rest between cycles, and you're well on your way.

Now, let's apply the HEGs to Hunter. Hunter needed to learn to read his tongue and eat fresher food. I taught him to use a tongue scraper—a small, metal, horseshoe-shaped instrument you can use to scrape the morning coating off your tongue—and a tongue map, which helps you read what appears on your tongue with regard to the state of your digestion and health of your organs. (You can find a printable tongue map in the *Body Thrive Workbook*). Because Hunter was a batch kind of guy, I taught him to make batches of sauerkraut. He experimented with fermenting various vegetables and spices. Fermented foods are packed with enzymes and turn up agni. I asked him to make fresh food at least every three days instead of once a week, which we both agreed he'd enjoy more. This is where we began.

As he made changes, Hunter's agni fired up and ama subsided. His tongue coating thinned. Once he streamlined his digestive energy he felt better, more energetic. His digestion improved, but not entirely. At a follow-up visit, we looked at what else was amiss. Hunter ate ice cream for dessert and cereal with milk in the morning. For breakfast, I asked him to switch to a hot grain cereal with almond milk or rice milk, and to replace the ice cream with gingersnaps most of the time. And, of course, I asked him to eat dinner earlier with dessert immediately following, and then to close his kitchen and brush his teeth.

With these additional changes, Hunter discovered he had a world of control over how he felt. When he slipped back and had ice cream instead of gingersnaps, his stomach felt crummy. He decided to cut out dairy entirely, and the rest of his ama disappeared. Hunter's bloating and stomach cramping days were over. He had more energy than he'd had in fifteen years.

If you have digestion, absorption, or elimination issues, you'll want to prioritize the HEGs over the other habits. The energy and time you invest here will empower you for the rest of your life. Digestion, absorption, and elimination should be smooth and pleasant. That is our target. These guidelines will help you get there.

Investigating the Healthier Eating Guidelines

The following three HEGs deserve special attention:

1. **Eat during daylight hours**   Our digestion evolved from our diurnal, pre-electricity era as humans. We liked to see our food, which we could only do by the light of the sun. We prepared food during the day so we wouldn't attract predators. As a result, our human bodies produce more bile, or digestive artillery, when the sun is high in the sky. Don't eat at night—leave three hours between your last meal and bedtime. If you're eating at night, go back to Habit 1, Eat an Earlier, Lighter Dinner. If you're wintering in the arctic, just make sure your big meal is during daylight.

2. **Be like Goldilocks**   This guideline is to fill your empty stomach with one-third food, one-third water, and one-third space, or room for digestion. Leave room for agni to churn and burn. That means not eating to fullness or stuffing yourself. When you stuff yourself, you steal energy for today and tomorrow. Do that repetitively for a few weeks and your stomach will stretch. Your sense of satiation will require more food, and you'll be in an endless cycle of stomach expansion.

   Stop the madness. Eat less. Use a smaller plate. Leave a few bites of food on your plate. Do whatever works for you to leave room for agni to churn and burn. Leave room for spirit, or your soul, to throw an after-dinner dance. Find other sources of pleasure instead of overeating—like a brisk walk after meals or a catnap following your midday meal.

3. **Take only water between meals**   Do you know what hunger feels like? Some of us put food to mouth throughout the day at the whim of our mind and emotions. I get it. I've been there. I used to eat little pieces of dark chocolate between meals. I also know, firsthand, that eating between meals, instead of drinking water or getting a breath of fresh air, is a terrific way to gain cellulite, waste bodily energy, and inculcate a scattered mind.

If you look closely at impulsive eating, you'll see it's habituated. There are triggers, habits, and rewards already at play, albeit unintentionally. When you see the pattern behind your actions—or the man behind the curtain—you can call your own bluff and put better triggers, habits, and rewards into place.

The hunger-satiation cycle is like the breath. You can't take a deep breath unless you're ready to be filled. You aren't ready to be filled until you're empty. You can't be empty if you're always inserting a little something into your piehole.

When you're truly hungry for a meal, your tongue is more accurate and your taste buds sharper. The meal didn't change. Your preparation to eat changed. Your senses were optimized to the experience of filling up, because your gut enjoyed being empty for a while.

When you eat before you're hungry, it doesn't taste as good. The digestive cycle gets overloaded and backed up, creating gas and bloating. You restock your blood sugar too quickly, so your body doesn't shift into fat metabolism. When you're metabolizing from your blood sugar, your thoughts and emotions are stressed, chaotic, intense, and negative. When you're in fat metabolism, your thoughts and emotions are stable, mellow, and positive. You design how you feel and think by how frequently you eat.

We often confuse hunger with thirst. The consequences of overeating far outweigh the consequences of overhydrating. The symptoms of dehydration (feeling low energy, dizzy, and cranky) mimic those of hunger. It's been estimated that 80 percent of our food cravings are thirst cravings in disguise. Before agriculture arose ten thousand years ago, we humans grazed on leaves, fruits, and stalks all day—in large part for hydration. When in doubt, drink water.

If you're truly hungry, you'll know in about twenty minutes with the chicken-scratching sensation in your breadbasket. Only food can satisfy true hunger. Thirst kicks in only after you're partially dehydrated. Again, when in doubt, apply the "yes, and" rule: Yes, I'm hungry, and I'd better drink a cup of water and wait a while to make sure it's really hunger.

Uprooting Outdated Cravings: An Intro to Detox

If you crave foods that work against your body, you have a disconnect. Your mind and your tongue are disconnected from what your bodily tissues desire. "Dumb" cravings are caused by ama. The ama acts like an evil imposter, taking over your emotions and your taste buds so that you crave and like that which generates more ama. You're trapped in a negative feedback loop.

The only escape route is detox. Ayurveda understands detox less as a broom and more like a fire. By giving agni space to burn, air to fan the flames, and lighter fluid to get sparky, the gunk in your cells gets incinerated. On a cellular level, agni gets sparked and incinerates the ama within or pushes the gunk back into circulation for removal via the poop, urine, menses, sweat, or snot.

To start detoxing, do less harm. Our bodies are astonishingly intelligent. A little cooperation is noted. Even before you start a "no" list, go with the "yes, and." Yes to green juice. Yes to vegetable soups. You won't have as much room for everything else. If you lighten your toxic load even a smidge today, by tomorrow less gunk goes into deeper tissue. Soon you feel better. You get curious about what a clean slate feels like.

There is also the deep-dive approach to detox. Even a short deep-dive detox—or quick immersion into what you should be doing—can efficiently lodge you in your new norm. When you emerge from a deep-dive detox, you're smarter, lighter, clearer, and less in denial about what doesn't work for you at this cycle in your life. You simultaneously reset your mind, your taste buds, your food-prep routine, and your menu-ordering habits.

Let go of the obvious, like alcohol, chocolate, coffee, smokes, crack, and processed food, along with wheat, meat, corn, and sugar for just a spell long enough to wipe the slate clean and smarten up your palate.

Within the world of detox, you have choices—fast or slow, intense or gentle, cooked or raw, whole foods or liquids, juices or soups. The basic idea is always the same: during a detox, you simplify what you take in through your five senses. You purify and rest. As you emerge, you nourish and protect your new foundling state of clarity, serenity, and purity.

Make your detox doable. As with any habit shift, you've got to want it, and you've got to feel competent you can execute. Doable detoxes, or system resets, should be done twice a year if there is physical or emotional ama or the desire to uplevel or retreat. (Consult the Do I Have Ama? checklist in the free *Body Thrive Workbook*.)

Eat the Six Tastes Daily

How you experience food depends on your five senses. The outer ecosystem becomes your inner ecosystem through your senses. Taste is the most obvious, as your body is fed nutrients to build bodily tissue through food. Your tongue has six sections to absorb the six tastes. All six of the tastes are needed for optimal digestion.

If you aren't eating all six tastes daily, your cravings will be off. If you don't include bitter, you may have excessive sweet cravings, as these opposites balance each other. The easiest way to integrate all six tastes in your day is at your midday meal.

The six tastes are sweet, sour, salty, pungent, bitter, and astringent. Each taste performs specific actions to design healthy functional tissues. Ayurveda codifies seven levels of tissue: plasma, blood, muscle, fat, bones, bone marrow, and procreation fluids. Good tissue formation of all seven tissues is a prerequisite for building ojas—deeply nutritive vitality, resilience, and immune integrity. Therefore, you need the six tastes to optimize immune function. The six tastes enhance the culture of the universe of you.

Moreover, if you leave out bitter, which refines and tightens the tissue, your cells will lack cohesion and tone. This is modeled in the Western diet, which lacks an abundance of dark, leafy greens and leads to obesity (a disease of excess building and lack of reduction).

Where to Find the Six Tastes

Bitter "Bitter is better," I've heard Dr. Lad say dozens of times. Bitter is the taste of dark, leafy greens. Sauté or lightly steam spinach, chard, kale, mustard greens, turnip greens, or dandelion greens. Dozens of different leafy greens are edible and have unique nutrient complexes. Diversify the greens in your salads, and add greens to smoothies.

Pungent Pungent is that spicy kick that breaks down heavier nutrients, releases stuck energy (including congestion), and increases circulation. Expand your spice repertoire, or simply start with a grind of fresh pepper or a cup of ginger tea. Certain greens, like mustard and arugula, and roots like radish or daikon, are strong in pungent taste.

Astringent Astringent helps your tissue pucker and firm up. A squeeze of fresh lemon juice or a side of beans is enough to indulge your astringent taste buds.

Sour Sour taste perks up your agni, enhances other flavors, and has a hydrophilic impact on your tissue. Fermented foods are the best way to get sour taste. A small scoop of homemade sauerkraut, a cup of miso soup, or a homemade yogurt sauce will meet your sour requirements.

Sweet Most likely you get plenty of sweet taste, which is anything that tastes nourishing. Grains, meats, breads, pasta, root vegetables, sweet fresh and dried fruits, and of course sweeteners of natural and artificial variety fall into this category. Notice that vegetables need to be divided into roots and greens. Roots are sweet and increase body weight; greens are bitter and decrease body weight. If you crave an excess of sweet, look to increase bitter.

Salty Salt enhances the appetite and enhances the other tastes. Use high-quality mineral salts and seaweed salts. If you have bloating or water retention, use a little less salt each day to rebalance your salty taste buds.

Review the list above, and add the missing tastes to that bigger, middle-of-the-day meal or very early dinner. The tastes, of course, are subject to the law of polarity. Like increases like, and the opposites reduce each other. The more you use hot sauce, the more hot sauce you'll crave. Same with salt and all the other tastes. Design your body by using the tastes that have the actions you want. Use the kaizen approach to add tastes that are missing from your meals. Add a slice of lemon to your green smoothie to incorporate astringent and sour taste, or shake in a dash of cinnamon to your cookie recipe for pungent taste. Read an Ayurvedic cookbook—my favorite is *The Everyday Ayurveda Cookbook: A Seasonal Guide to Eating and Living Well* by Kate O'Donnell—to develop your abilities to optimize the six tastes in your meals and give your body what it needs.

With practice, your palate won't let you leave out a taste. As your palate smartens up, you are less likely to use your sense of taste poorly, thus averting the second cause of disease. Furthermore, you'll be more attracted to the tastes that are seasonally dominant and prevent seasonal imbalances that would contribute to the third cause of disease—living out of sync with the cosmic clock.

Personal Calamities with the HEGs

By my teen years, I had snot regardless of the season. My dad nicknamed me "Foghorn." Running out of tissues at high school frequently led to classroom calamities. My doctor proclaimed the cause to be allergies.

From the Ayurvedic perspective, the cause was ama, which is often a major factor in allergies and other immune disorders where you react to your ecosystem. I grew up violating the quintessential Ayurvedic habit by eating a late dinner, often with ice cream for dessert.

As a young adult studying Ayurveda, I did an experiment to see if my allergies were caused by my choices or my ecosystem. I detoxed with Ayurvedic *kitchari* (meaning a mixture of grains), a rice and mung-bean stew, and the standard home *panchakarma* (Ayurvedic cleansing) practices for seven days. I administered *nasya*, an Ayurvedic detox therapy where you snort warm, herbal oil that is designed for your particular imbalances. Snot flowed out of me profusely for two weeks. After the blowout, the snot was gone. All of it. Gone. In fourteen days. Afterward, I had no need for drugs or tissues.

My first detox was a challenge, but the detox itself turned out to be the easy part. The hard part was saying no to ice cream after the detox. This is where *asatmendriyartha samyoga*—disrespecting your senses—came in big time. There is an effort, a tapas, that appears with transformation. If that effort demands too much discipline all at once, you fail. I failed. I'm embarrassed to admit that soon after my transforming detox, I was eating a pint of Ben & Jerry's ice cream. My cognitive maturity was way ahead of my emotional maturity. The snot returned.

Bulldozing a bad habit is harder than constructing a good habit. I could have applied "yes, and" and had a spoon of raw honey and a cup of ginger tea after dinner. Then if I still wanted ice cream, I would be appeased by less. Shift your focus from uprooting a negative habit to feeding a better habit.

After years, I transcended the ice-cream-to-snot pattern. I added the habit of detoxing every six months. My tongue grew smarter as I became ama-free and wanted nutrients, not filler. Slowly but surely, my palate matured.

When you engage a time perspective on your own samskaras and how deep their nocuous roots grow, you can collaborate with yourself and nurture a cooperative approach to their dissolution. Be honest with what you *should* do and what you *can* do now. Add a small, doable habit. You'll avoid subtly beating yourself up for your lack of integrity when your willpower fails.

Limiting Beliefs and Healthier Eating Guidelines

Below I share the Limiting Beliefs/Higher Truths tool, which helps reveal the undercurrents of self-sabotage. I wish I'd had this tool back in my ice-cream-to-snot days.

On the left side, write any beliefs around the habits you have that you know aren't getting you what you want in the long run. For example, "I'm an emotional eater." Then, pause. Reflect. Dig up the higher, more updated version of the truth. This is your deeper truth. In this example, "I go through phases of emotional eating," is a deeper truth. Below, you can see from examples how to use an unhealthy consistent craving to unpack your behind-the-scenes assumptions.

Limiting Belief	Higher Truth
I don't have time to exercise.	I could take a five-minute walk after dinner.
Ice cream is so satisfying.	Ice cream isn't as satisfying as it used to be.
Food is a good reward.	I can think of better rewards that won't sabotage my body.
I don't have time to eat healthy.	I need to learn how to prepare healthy food. I should hire a coach to help me.
One glass of wine at night is good for me.	One glass often turns into two. My sleep is often disturbed. I feel groggy in the morning.

You're not conscious of your limiting beliefs or higher truths until you take the time to investigate them. Take the time to reflect and write down what is more true now. You need to see this on paper. Fill in the Limiting Beliefs/Higher Truths worksheet in the *Body Thrive Workbook* at bodythrive.com/free. You'll discover the deeper, updated version of the truth. What you find will surprise you and bring your actions into integrity with your beliefs.

The Anti-Fad Way to Eat

When I first learned the HEGs, most of them were *not* my current habits. I jogged during lunch hour and afterward ate a light salad at my desk while working. I snacked. I had no idea about the six tastes or eating to fill the stomach one-third with food, one-third with water, and one-third with space, or room, for digestion. I didn't know my eating habits generated allergies, weight gain, a poor body image, and acne. Now, after fifteen years, these guidelines are in my back pocket. Though I rebelled against each of them, slowly I built momentum.

The HEGs are controversial from the perspective of allopathic nutrition. Your doctor may advise you to eat six small meals a day to lose weight. Ayurveda would rather you digest completely and rest between meals for maximum bodily and mental agility.

Ayurvedic eating is the anti-fad diet, hanging in the background for thousands of years. Ayurveda at its most basic is folk medicine: grandmother kitchen wisdom.

My French grandmother liked to suck the marrow out of her lamb chops. She'd snag the bones that I rejected, informing me it was the best part. From an Ayurvedic perspective, she was right. The bone marrow is the most complex, nutrient-dense tissue in that chop. My Polish grandmother taught me the little I know about eating organ meat. I learned a chopped liver recipe from her. Liver, it turns out, is in the top ten most nutrient-dense foods on the planet.

Ayurveda has been cultivated in a culture of lactovegetarians. No chicken liver. Lots of ghee replacing the bone marrow. Adapt the teachings of Ayurveda to your own ancestry and ecosystem.

The Kitchen Sadhana chapter on page 213 offers some suggestions that will get you plugged into your ancestral taste buds.

Ayurveda is obsessed with digestion because imbalanced digestion is the root of most body-mind imbalances. Have you eaten when upset and noticed your belly couldn't handle the food? You marry what you eat with the emotions you experience while eating.

In Ayurvedic diagnostics, we look at a person's unique constitution and the nature of their imbalance. We investigate the type of agni. "Hangry" (or irritable when hungry) indicates sharp agni. Skipping meals and eating in an unpredictable pattern indicates sporadic agni. A sluggish, heavy gut indicates slow agni. No problems whatsoever, coupled with a pleasant demeanor, indicates *sama agni*. The HEGs help all types move toward balanced digestion and a pleasant demeanor.

Eating for your constitution is a high priority if you have digestive issues. Take a constitutional quiz at bodythrive.com/quiz.

Marry Your Foods Wisely

You want to marry your foods with your constitution and digestive type. In general, if you have sporadic mealtimes, get on a schedule. If you bloat when you eat, start to eat one-pot meals. Choose dishes that are soupy, warm, well spiced, and have high-quality fats. If you get hangry, eat on schedule, eat more protein and a little fat with each meal, and *stop snacking*. With this regimen, blood sugar usually stabilizes within ten days. If you have slow digestion, eat just twice a day, around 10:00 a.m. and 4:00 p.m., and spice up your dishes.

What you eat combines in the pot, on the plate, and eventually in your belly. Certain foods enhance digestion when combined. Others throw jabs and hooks in your gut. The physical experience in your gut directly influences your mental-emotional experience as the food works its way into you and through you. As many an elder has advised, marry wisely.

Here are the major Ayurvedic rules for food combining. The more sensitive your gut, the less you want to break the rules.

- Raw fruit should be taken alone or with greens. Otherwise it causes other foods to ferment in your gut, and you'll bloat. If you want raw fruit, eat it thirty minutes before the rest of your meal. Fruit with granola and yogurt for breakfast is enough to overwork your gut for an entire day. A green smoothie with just fruit and greens is easy to digest, but if you add nut milks and protein powder—good luck.

- No milk with meals. Milk is best taken warmed, spiced, and alone. It's heavy and difficult to digest. A little in oatmeal or rice pudding may be fine for you.

- Yogurt only combines with vegetables and grains.

- Eggs only combine with nonstarchy vegetables and grains.

- Beans only combine with grains, greens, roots, other beans, and nuts and seeds, not eggs, cheese, or meat.

Remember, the more energy you want to have, the more you need to lighten the workload in your gut. If you have digestive issues and you notice that you're breaking the food-combining rules, start with awareness. If you eat yogurt with granola, notice if you get bloated or gassy. Always start with awareness, notice cause and effect, and then plan ahead for what you'll have instead next time. Get an Ayurvedic cookbook—the recipes will combine food properly.

TIPS FOR HEALTHIER EATING

- Use the worksheets in the *Body Thrive Workbook*.

- Dial in one HEG at a time. Start with this easy one: enjoy your food and really taste it. The HEGs interconnect. Soon, you'll find you prefer the guidelines.

- Notice cause and effect. When you disregard a guideline, notice the effects. Trace back your symptoms to the offense. Be brutally honest, because karma doesn't lie.

- If you're a chronic snacker, add short bursts of exercise, drinking water, and deep breathing between meals. Soon, you'll love the mental clarity and emotional steadiness that comes from metabolizing fat.

- If you have ama, do a detox. Yogidetox.com goes live online every April and October. Join us—we rock the detox.

- If you usually overeat, have a pint of water twenty minutes before eating.

- Use the Limiting Beliefs/Higher Truths worksheet in the *Body Thrive Workbook*.

- Learn about the six tastes in Ayurvedic food preparation. If you aren't incorporating them all, learn from an Ayurvedic cookbook.

Come to Your Senses

WHAT TO DO

Learn the basics and enable your senses to last a lifetime. Each sense organ has specific, self-care therapies and practices. Know your weaknesses and start using those therapies.

WHY YOU WANT TO DO IT

We all want to hear, see, smell, and taste well as we get older. Don't let your sense organs devitalize prematurely.

HOW TO START

Pick one of the self-care suggestions in this chapter. Schedule it. Build it into your daily routine. Start with something simple, like scraping your tongue or lubing your nostrils. Most of these protective rituals take seconds daily, yet they pay off big both day-to-day and in old age.

Take a moment and think about what your senses do for you. Imagine life without sight. Without hearing. Without the sense of touch. Without taste. Without smell. Your senses are the gateway to what you perceive. What you perceive, you experience.

No one wants to lose their senses. Hearing can fade. Eyes can lose their focus and end up behind glasses. Skin wrinkles and roughens. Taste and smell lose their acuity. As this happens, the world you sense becomes smaller. And although technology is improving, anyone with a hearing aid—even one that's state of the art—will let you know it's not as good as the real thing, baby. This chapter is a crash course in optimizing your senses for acuity now and longevity later.

Sense organ habits are not usually keystone habits, which anchor and trigger other habits. Sense organ habits are simple, fast, and require little discipline or motivation. Stack them onto habits that you've already dialed in around bedtime, waking, and mealtime.

Getting Fat and Visually Impaired

Working with Cicely, I witnessed how diet affects eyesight. When I met her, she was newly certified as a yoga teacher, thirty years young and about fifty pounds overweight. The weight came on during high school, when her father left home and her mother went to work. After fourteen years of carrying extra weight—and needing stronger eyeglass prescriptions—Cicely chose to change.

She joined Yogidetox, and the weight began to fall off. She joined the Living Ayurveda Course to surround herself with healthy, supportive people and continued guidance. With this support, the fat continued to melt.

Cicely hoped the weight loss would improve her overall health. But over time, her eyeglasses stopped working. Disappointed, she went to the doctor. At the eye doctor's office, she was shocked to learn that her glasses didn't work because her eyes were improving.

Slowly, Cicely worked her way backward through her old eyeglass prescriptions as her vision rapidly regenerated over the following year. Her poor eating habits had affected her vision. When Cicely analyzed the cost of her prescription glasses over the past decade of weight gain, she realized her new habits would save her buckets of money.

The rate at which wear and tear of your body occurs is under your control. How your senses age depends on how you use them and what you choose for your senses to merge with, which influences what you think and feel. Use your habits to come to your senses.

Protect Your Senses

Your senses are the gateways to experience the world. Think about it. When you talk about an experience, analyze your words to discover which senses you rely on the most. For example: "Yesterday, I had a spectacular mountain bike ride through the forest. The trees and birds were singing, the wildflowers grew as tall as my head, and the meadows were thick with that moist, luscious fragrance."

You want to protect your senses to perceive the world accurately, fully, and delightfully as you age. Otherwise, there will be grime on the windshield of your perception. When your sense gateways and mind are clear, you're more in touch with reality and connected to your community.

Specific practices lengthen the life span of your senses. Each sense organ has a few therapies that, when done daily, can heal damage now or prevent problems later. As you read through this chapter, identify which practices will help you the most and are the easiest to integrate into other habits.

Print the sense-organ tip sheets and charts from the *Body Thrive Workbook* (bodythrive.com/free), and tape them where you'll use them. For instance, tape the tongue chart to the bathroom mirror, at eye level. Tape the eye exercise worksheet near your computer, or use it as a bookmark if you read a lot.

Don't Brush Your Tongue—Scrape It

You already know your tongue is in charge of what you spit or swallow. To start optimizing your sense of taste, you need two things:

- A stainless-steel tongue scraper; you can get it from Banyan Botanicals or search online. You can start with using a spoon to do the job, but it won't match up to a $10 tongue scraper that will last the rest of your life.

- A tongue chart

First thing in the morning, before you drink your quart of water, scrape your tongue from back to front seven to fourteen times. Then, look at the gunk you pulled onto your tongue scraper. It is light and clear? If so, good. Is it thick, white, and chunky? If so, not so good. That is ama. If you have ama on your tongue scraper, look at a tongue chart and see exactly where the ama is collecting in your gut. Is it in your stomach? Your small intestine? Your colon? Go on an ama hunt.

After you scrape, look at your tongue. Is it healthy pink? Patchy? White? Pale? Greasy? Dry? Inflamed? Do you have scallops along the sides? Cracks? Read your tongue using the tongue chart on page 183. Read your friends' tongues to notice differences and signs of imbalance. It's fun. Your tongue mirrors your digestion, the states of your nervous system, and your organ health. Your tongue is a microcosm, a hologram, of the universe of you.

Once you've self-diagnosed and scraped your tongue, take a moment to reflect. Remember that as the ambassador for the body, the tongue signals what's needed. If your tongue had any symptoms on the chart, what could you do differently today to take better care of yourself? If you had a thick white coating, gently scrape off what is easily scrapeable, then drink some ginger tea ASAP and throughout the day. Eat light, warm, and spicy foods, like lentil soup. The white coating on your tongue indicates your stomach has excess mucus. If you were to eat a bagel and cream cheese that might be enough to overwhelm your body, resulting in a cold or flu. By noticing the thick, white coating in the morning you can make choices to harmonize your digestion and avoid getting sick.

As your tongue becomes healthier, notice how your cravings and sense of taste wise up. Refined sugars will have a bitter, dead aftertaste and leave your mouth feeling icky. Wild foods will taste vibrant, crazy, and leave your mouth feeling clean. You'll stop swallowing food that doesn't give your tongue a "Hell, yeah!"

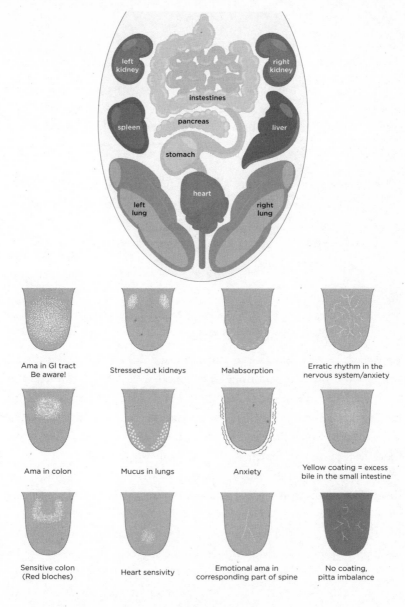

Ama in GI tract
Be aware!

Stressed-out kidneys

Malabsorption

Erratic rhythm in the
nervous system/anxiety

Ama in colon

Mucus in lungs

Anxiety

Yellow coating = excess
bile in the small intestine

Sensitive colon
(Red bloches)

Heart sensivity

Emotional ama in
corresponding part of spine

No coating,
pitta imbalance

Ayurvedic Tongue Chart

Get to know your tongue by printing this chart and taping it
to your bathroom mirror. Do you have a healthy, pink tongue?
Or do you have patches, cracks, bumps, or different colors?
As you get to know your tongue you'll notice subtle changes.
You can track your tongue's evolution back to a healthy,
even pink color as you refine your Body Thrive Habits.

TIPS TO OPTIMIZE TASTE

- Get a metal tongue scraper.

- Print your tongue chart and tape it near your bathroom mirror.

- Scrape your tongue first thing in the morning, *before* drinking water. Then, taste the quality of your water.

- Use the blank tongue charts in the workbook to diagnose your tongue.

Eyes: You Are What You See

Your eyes are very sensitive to stress, tension, and fatigue of any kind, whether it's physical, emotional, or mental. When the eyes focus and are pulled forward in the socket, they strain. Many of you have heard the instruction in yoga class to soften your eyes, even in the face of an intense pose. In softening your eyes, you relax your nerves and allow fluids to cleanse and replenish the eye tissue for longevity.

As I type, I feel my eyes get tired. What to do? I make a choice. Instead of ignoring the message from my eyes, I raise and soften my gaze. I find a window where I can see the sky, or I step outside. I let my eyes diffuse on the horizon. Anyone who works on a computer or reads a lot should do this multiple times a day.

Balance comes down to attending to the opposites. If you use your eyes to focus, integrate a habit that allows your gaze to diffuse. Otherwise, you'll wear out your eyes early in life and still have decades to live. Another tip: if you stare at a screen for most of your day, put a plant on or near your desk, allow your eyes to rest on a plant's green color. Human eyes are restored by the cooling, harmonizing vibration of living green color. Take "gazing" breaks every thirty minutes for at least thirty seconds.

If you have tired eyes, lie on your back and place an eye bag over your eyes. An eye bag is best filled with flaxseeds—soft, oily seeds that provide the perfect weight and texture for allowing the eyeballs to release backward and away from the dry air and into the sockets where fluids circulate, nourish, and replenish. If you don't have an eye bag, rub your palms together and palm your eyes. Try one of these practices now, and notice the effects.

TIPS FOR LIFELONG VISION

- Do the exercises on the Eye Care Practices Worksheet, including palming, focusing, and flexing your eyes.

- Rest your eyes on the horizon after periods of reading or concentration.

- Rest with an eye bag to release unconscious tension before bed.

- Maintain your body's ideal weight.

- Glasses and contacts don't address the underlying pattern that produced and perpetuates the vision problem. Work with a holistic vision specialist.

- When practicing yoga, relax your eyes. When conversing, relax your eyes. When reading, relax your eyes. When driving, relax your eyes and pay attention.

- Learn about *netra basti* if you have tired, dry eyes. It's a blissful therapy that involves bathing your eyes in clarified butter. You can see an Ayurvedic practitioner or try the do-it-yourself version.

- Sit in silence and rest your gaze.

Replenish Your Hearing

Your ears are always listening. They work via vibration. Vibration requires space and movement through that space. The best way to replenish the ears and balance their expansive nature is to fill them with warm oil. The therapy is called *karna purana*. Once a month, take ten minutes to nourish your ears. I warm a one-ounce dropper bottle of sesame oil by placing it in a teacup filled with body-temperature water. Then, lying comfortably on my side, with my head supported by an old towel, I fill the ear that's turned toward the ceiling with the warm oil. I relax. After a few minutes, I slowly roll over, pouring the oil from my ear into a shallow bowl. Placing a cotton ball in that ear, I repeat on the other side.

The quick-and-easy daily version goes like this: when you get out of the shower, dry your face and ears. Put a few drops of sesame or coconut oil on your middle fingers. Insert into outer ear holes, about half an inch. Make rapid circles with your index fingers, gently lubricating and stretching the inner ears.

Throughout your day, notice the sounds that make you thrive. Just like you are what you eat, you are what you hear. Listen to the voices that attract you. Spend more time with those people. Pay attention. Listen to the sounds in nature that attract you—is it running water or the rustling of leaves? Respect the delicate nature of your hearing. What sounds align with who you want to become?

TIPS TO PROLONG YOUR HEARING

- Trust your ears—avoid loud, aggressive, or harsh sounds.

- When listening, listen deeply. When you've had your fill, find silence.

- Take in the sounds of nature. You can do this as a listening meditation.

- When your hearing is overly sensitive, use the oil-in-the-ears therapy described below.

- For tinnitus, or if you're a light sleeper, try sleeping with oily cotton balls in your ears—wet side in. Use sesame oil.

- Balance sound with silence.

Don't Pick Your Nose—Lube It

Your nostrils are the primary pathway for life force to enter your body. Through nostril breathing (not mouth breathing), prana accesses the lower lobes of your lungs, which activates your body's natural relaxation response. When in doubt or stressed out, breathe through your nostrils into the lower part of your rib cage.

Dry nostrils lead to dry sinuses, which lead to an ineffective air filtration system. If your nostrils are dry, they can't catch unwanted pathogens, germs, or microbes. The germs pass unnoticed into the universe of you, embedding in deeper tissue; wreaking havoc with your lungs, throat, and sinuses; and turning into infections, colds, or the flu. Keeping your nostrils clear and lubricated prevents sickness while enabling you to absorb more oxygen.

Following the pattern of oil and orifices, you may guess that Ayurveda is big on nostril lubing. As dry skin gets lubed, it functions like an effective filter. Of all the bodily orifices, the nostrils, which are constantly passing air, dry out most. I can just hear the postmenopausal vata women out there saying a different hole is drier. In any case, love your nostrils with a good daily greasing.

Bonus: Teach your kids to love their nostrils with lube, too. When your kids lube their nostrils, snot won't collect, so they won't pick.

- Keep a small jar of coconut oil or ghee next to the sink where you brush your teeth. Use your pinky finger to apply oil in circular motions inside your nostrils.

- Or, use a nasya oil or Yogahealer's Sinus Lube. Snort a few drops or up to half an eyedropper of oil into each nostril, each morning. Spit out any that comes through to your mouth. The essential oils open your senses.

Tips to Save Time

Many of the sense-organ self-care habits can happen all at once. When you're doing your self-massage, rub the oil in your ears and nostrils. Take a moment and palm your eyes. There, you hit all four in a matter of minutes, and if you scraped your tongue before your morning water, you've hit sense-care proficiency. You've lubed your skin, ears, and nostrils. You've scraped your tongue. You've relaxed your eyes. Take a moment in silence to rest in your senses. You've come to your senses.

If You Love It, Oil It: Apply Anywhere

In Ayurveda, we have a very simple formula for loving and protecting the body. The formula is this: to increase love and protection, rub in oil.

When I graduated from both the Ayurveda College and the Yoga Institute in 2001, I wanted to teach a workshop named "Oil and Orifices." I talked to a few yoga studios about the class, and we determined the yoga studios of San Francisco weren't ready for this . . . yet. But you can find the Oil and Orifices for Self-Massage worksheet in the *Body Thrive Workbook*.

Fast-forward fifteen years—we're ready. How many holes do you have in your body? Go ahead. Count how many holes are in the universe of you. Two nose holes, two ear holes, one piehole, two eye sockets, two tear ducts, one poop hole, one pee hole, sweat ducts, one belly button (at one point it was a real hole), two nipples, and for women, one baby-making/baby-ejecting hole. These are the many points of entry and exit for herbs and oils to heal, soothe, and detox the body.

You may swish oil in your mouth to loosen gunk and protect teeth (oil pulling), soak your tired eyes in pools of ghee (netra basti therapy), insert a coconut-oil-saturated tampon to counter vaginal dryness, use oil enemas to calm anxiety. You name it, Ayurveda has an oil, an herb, and an orifice for it. Thinking of your points of entry and exit will help you experiment with your body to make better choices through what you take in and what you release.

You use the law of polarity to find balance. If your nostrils are usually clogged with thick mucus, using a saltwater neti-pot rinse will help open the channels. Drinking a tea of sage and black pepper will heat you up and dry you out. However, if your mucus is thin and your nostrils and lungs feel dry, you'll want to use nasal oil and drink a demulcent tea, like licorice root and fennel.

How to Lose Your Senses

For those who want to see how the senses are intricately tied into disease, pay attention. Otherwise, skip ahead to Habit 10: Live in Ease. Here is a refresher on the three causes of disease:

- *Prajnaparadha*: Making negligent choices
- *Asatmendriyartha samyoga*: Disrespecting your senses
- *Parinama*: Living out of rhythm

Prajnaparadha is triggered whenever you know better but fail to employ what you have learned. You strengthen the pattern of imbalance, which diminishes sensory acuity. Eventually, the sense dulls out, unable to do its job, and your world gets a little smaller as your perceptivity shrinks.

With asatmendriyartha samyoga, you overuse, misuse, neglect, or abuse your senses. Overuse of the eyes occurs when you continue to stare at a computer even after your eyes feel tired. If you do this daily, you'll get headaches and need glasses. Misuse of your tongue happens when you crave potato chips and eat the whole bag. Abuse of your ears happens at loud concerts and in subway stations.

Your senses guide and protect your biochemistry. If you neglect your senses, you contract your biochemistry and your perception. Your senses are attuned by an exacting desire. Just enough sweet taste is good for you. Just enough visual and mental stimulation is A-OK. When you push the envelope too far, you don't just damage a sense organ, you place undue stress on your entire operating system.

Use your senses just right. They're exquisite, and your tastes develop with age. Respect your organs, and as you age you'll perceive more, not less.

Next time you're eating a meal, notice when it becomes less pleasurable. Notice the exact moment when your body has had enough. Listen. Respect. Obey. Your senses will sharpen from your smart decision, ready to receive exquisite experiences tomorrow.

There is a touch of the inevitable with parinama, or regular wear and tear over time. And yet . . . there is leeway.

Parinama and Seasonal Respites to Recharge the Senses

While parinama may seem inevitable, you can activate the seasons and cycles of time to advance your health. This is the topic of *ritucharya*, or optimizing seasonal rhythms.

Seasons are marked by junctures—which are moments of opportunity for wellness evolution. Seasonal cleansing, or biannual detox, extends your life by taking out your inner trash. The trash, in this case, is any seasonal buildup of the doshas or ama. At the end of summer, you probably have a buildup of heat in your blood and liver. At the end of fall, you probably have a buildup of dryness in your lymph, colon, and nerves. At the end of winter, you probably have a buildup of cold and stagnation in your lymph, lungs, and fat. At the end of spring, you probably have a buildup of damp and cool qualities in your lymph and stomach.

Around and around you go. When you stop nobody knows.

Yet how you go around, and when you empty the buckets of your imbalances, is in your own hands. Most of us weren't raised with this "empty your bucket" body wisdom, so you don't know which of the symptoms of aging are optional.

If you allow the doshas to build up and overflow, season to season, they move from superficial tissue (like from the GI tract through the lymph, blood, and muscle tissue) into your deeper tissues, senses, organs, and systems. Imbalances, or dis-ease, turn into disease, as they embed deeper into the body and cause dysfunction. The deeper these imbalances move, the more qualitative disruption occurs in the tissue system they are affecting. Or so goes the Ayurvedic theory of pathogenesis.

For example, heat built up from summer may present as a skin rash in June, irritability in July, vocational burnout in August, a sinus infection in October, and strep throat after the holidays. If this pattern is kept up year after year, you might have shingles next season.

When you use the change of seasons to dump off imbalanced doshas (like the excess pitta in the above example) through a detox, you upgrade your body's operating system. You can release physical as well as emotional ama. Season by season, you can wake up wiser. With your senses alert and refreshed, you perceive the world more accurately and on a subtler plane. Renewed and rejuvenated, you make better choices.

I've heard a thousand Yogidetoxers report how their senses wake up. Eyesight improves, hearing improves, skin and sense of touch improve, the tongue can taste more accurately, the nose becomes alert like that of a canine.

The lesson here is simple. If you don't discover the power of seasonal detox, you'll create wear and tear on your senses faster. Even with the season-by-season aging process, you have opportunities to advance your wellness. Ritucharya teaches us to respect the beautiful intersections where time and space open to help us heal and begin anew. Pay attention when change is in the air.

HABIT 10

Live in Ease

WHAT TO DO

When you notice stress, choose ease. The problem isn't the problem. Your reaction to the problem is the problem. Stabilize your day-to-day perspective in the expanded backdrop of easeful awareness; be in touch with intrinsic plenitude.

WHY YOU WANT TO DO IT

Like a toggle switch in your nervous system, you live in either reaction or reception. The first perpetuates stress; the latter cultivates ease. One unconsciously meanders toward unconscious tension, limitation, and disconnection. The other intentionally leads to an extraordinary, heart-centric, intimate, and evolutionary life.

Allow stress, overwhelm, or anxiety to fade into the background as you focus on living into what each day unfurls. You'll enjoy an extraordinary life and become an inspired leader for your future.

Return to these simple touch-points throughout your day: Receive the gift of breath. Receive the earth beneath you. Receive the heavens above. Receive a drink of water. Receive the gift of the company you keep. Relax and enjoy your senses. Your senses situate you in the present. Orient your senses to receive. Look for beauty. Listen for wisdom. Speak with connection. Touch with sensitivity. Now, allow your awareness to expand, infinitely, beyond yourself. Situate your perspective to expanded, interconnected awareness.

You become a gift to others through being awake, connected, and reflecting the intrinsic blessing of life. You can become increasingly available to the minute and massive gifts of life if you adopt the habit of an easeful, interconnected perspective. Situated in expanded awareness, you become available to the evolutionary unfolding of the now interfacing with the future.

The other nine habits slowly and simultaneously give rise to the habit of Live in Ease. If this habit evades you, start with the others. Then, bit by bit, when you notice stress, flip the switch to ease. You always have a choice.

Are You Choosing Stress or Ease?

Find out where you are on the spectrum between ease and stress. See how many statements apply to you from the lists below. Take a breath. Be honest, and you'll uplevel your integrity.

Do you orient from stress?

- You are overwhelmed.

- You wake up feeling rushed into your day.

- You often wish you were doing something else.

- You're pressed for time, and often show up late.

- Your body feels heavy and sluggish in the morning.

- You feel trapped in your life or your body.

- You want to make changes, but it seems too difficult.

- You're wired, but tired, and you wish you could sleep through the night uninterrupted.

- You're depressed by the people in your life.

Do you orient from ease?

- You wake up in joy.

- You work hard and give life your all.

- Your life is on purpose, with time for reflection and course correction.

- You're inspired by the people in your life.

- You spend time daily in silence, inquiry, or quiet reflection.

- Others experience you as grounded, interesting, and inspiring.

- Your relationships are deeply honest, in integrity, intimate, and future oriented.

- You lead when a situation calls for leadership.

- You often find yourself tapped into a timeless, spacious experience, both when alone and when with loved ones.

Alchemizing Ease

This final essential habit, Live in Ease, is about alchemizing ease. Easeful living is defined by how you orient your awareness and what that perpetuates. This habit awakens the power to shift from victim to victor, from passive to active, from reactionary to evolutionary. You want to upgrade the default mode of your perspective throughout your day.

At every core, you find a seed. At the deep core of every human, you find the seed of orientation. Will it toggle toward stress or ease? Each human has the power to choose. Half full or half empty? Poison or panacea? Contract or expand? The choice is yours, moment by moment, day by day, year by year, decade by decade. You can alchemize the poison of stress into the elixir of ease.

Embracing the Friction of Evolutionary Tension

You were raised, culturally speaking, on existential tension. Tension is contractive, tightening, hardening, and a necessary component of evolution. In the law of polarity, its opposite or dynamic variable is expansion. As like increases like, when you unconsciously operate from tension, you feel separate, stressed, and subtly discontented. And if you are unaware, you won't even notice your experience of being separate or discontented—it feels normal—and the contraction continues.

You can choose expansion even when tension is present. You can train your awareness. You can build a habit to expand your perspective, to orient to the ground of being, which is nonlocal to your body or mind. You can cultivate a bigger perspective beyond local time and space, which relaxes your nerves and enlarges your sense of self and interconnectivity. It is not about living in a self-absorbed, blissed-out state. Easeful living is about showing up every day on purpose, in action, from a connected, open inner space.

Anytime you decide to become more, you can expect a rub. The yogis call the friction of transformation *tapas*. Though a predictable part of the path of awakening, tapas is never comfortable. In his "Principles of Evolutionary Culture," Craig Hamilton writes "If we're not uncomfortable, we're probably not evolving."[1]

As your habits evolve, tension will arise. The challenge you face in growth is naturally intimidating and just too much at times. The existential battle is on for the old self versus the emerging self. Expect struggle, setbacks, shadows, confusion, disorientation, and distractions.

Easeful living makes it possible to operate from a bigger perspective as the going gets tough. This mindset balances out the fear of failure, fear of the unknown, and fear of incompetence with a willingness, a miracle-mindedness, and an opportunity orientation. Stress can roll like water off a duck's back. We're able to become a bigger, better version of ourselves.

This is a newer skill on humanity's timeline. You are breaking free of a more primitive, reactive, self-centered, or overwhelmed culture. You are building the habit of being receptive, open to possibility, even when you're unsure or afraid.

I'm Nothing but You

The fabulous Tantric scholar Dr. Douglas Brooks teaches, "I'm not you; I'm not like you; I'm nothing but you."[2] This statement reflects the fundamental teaching of nonduality, where unity consciousness and separation consciousness coexist. As we all have the faculty for both, we can cultivate facility with both. Separation consciousness is something most of us don't have a problem accessing. The friction is in stabilizing awareness in the whole of creation.

"The Tantrics begin with a spiritual paradigm," says Brooks. "'I'm not you; I'm not like you; I'm nothing but you.' Think about that: 'I'm not you,' because we're different people. 'I'm not like you,' because we think and feel and understand the world in different ways. But 'I'm nothing but you,' because we're all part of the same creation. How can that be? That's what you try to understand when you study religion."[3]

You can develop a habit of interconnecting your perspective. You start to see the other as the self. Your mind opens, and you become available for conscious connection. Some perceive it as the gateway of surrendering the small self to become part of the larger whole. Many are convinced this perspective is imperative for a brighter future for us all. This expanded vantage point orients you to inclusivity and empathy. You reestablish interconnectivity, bridging the gap of separation, transforming stress into A-OK-ness. Identifying as the whole of creation while simultaneously being an independent actor able to influence the creation is what this is about. Going from feeling separate to feeling part of the whole turns stress into ease.

Receive Your Natural State

Another term for the same creation we're all a part of is the "ground of being." When you uproot, you lose your receptivity to the ground of being. You get trapped, unconsciously, in the viewpoint of limitation and lack. Uprooted, your actions, thoughts, and even your emotions shift. Operating under the illusion of separation, you turn away from intimate connection and depth. You repeat your past. Yogis call the illusion of separation *maya*, or the veil, and the repeating of the past *samskara*.

Right behind the façade of stress is the subtle backdrop of expanded awareness. Under your insecurities is your competence. The stress mindset causes you to forget that you are whole, that you are A-OK in this moment. Then, you compete instead of collaborate. You construct obstacles instead of creating collaborative solutions. Yet your expanded awareness is always right here, not even a breath away.

Easeful living is a grounded connection to your natural state, your divine inheritance as a human, and the basic teachings of heaven on earth. Three Sanskrit words—*purna, sukha*, and *dukha*—perhaps can help hack the simplicity of this subtle habit.

You will recall that purna (purnatva) means "intrinsic fullness," referring to the full moon, our true state. At any other moon cycle, you misconstrue the shape of the moon based on what is visible. The moon is lit by the sun. Your inner fullness is lit by the light of being. If you don't contract, the light shines through you, uplifting others.

However separate you feel obscures that same amount of light from shining through, like during a crescent moon.

Easeful living can also be understood by the teachings of sukha and dukha. *Sukha* is ease. *Dukha* is suffering. They share the root *kha*, which means "ether" (*akasha*)—the space in which everything arises, including us.

What is the quality of your inner space where your thoughts and emotions are circulating? What is the quality of the space between us? *Sukha* means the space is clean, clear—nothing obscures your connection to expanded awareness. You shine. Inversely, *dukha* means the space is dirty, obscured; suffering arises because you're operating under the misperception of feeling separate and lonely.

The Yoga Sutras also help us understand the power of easeful living with the teaching *Sthira Sukham Asanam*, which I interpret as "Awakening arises from a steady, easeful orientation." The Sanskrit word *asanam* means your "seat," or the posture from which we orient our life. As the first word in the sutra, *sthira* (meaning "steady") is the starting point. *Sukham* means "ease," which relies on "clean space." It's the opposite of *dukha*, which means "suffering" and "dirty space." As you live the 10 Habits of Body Thrive, your cells will have less congestion, less toxicity, and more coordinated rhythm, which arise from clarified space. This creates a daily experience of steady ease.

Sthira Sukham Asanam is your potential mode of daily orientation—relaxed and alert. Contrast this with the experience of rushing from one action to the next, harried, disgruntled, and tired. How do you practice shifting your orientation to life? What are the steps?

The Other Habits and Easeful Living

You get access to Live in Ease through the other nine habits compounding over time. Conversely, if you blow off the other habits, you barricade the door to easeful living. If you aren't early to bed, you won't be rested to rise early for the predawn, deep, etheric fullness. If you eat dinner too late, you'll be full of partially digested food and waste, and you won't have access to the spaciousness of being. If you haven't carved out space to start the day right or for meditation, this habit will be out of reach.

The habits of Start Your Day Right and Sit in Silence drill you to surrender your egoic nature and open to a larger perspective. The problem is that you get on with your day and forget. A few hours later, you notice you're not in ease. You're in stress. Perhaps you've created a pressure cave by trying to get more done than is possible in the allotted time. Perhaps, agitated from lack of sleep, you hear your own voice speaking to your child in a way that doesn't reflect your deeper wisdom. Perhaps, due to a strong emotional pattern, you place awareness on the outdated thoughts and outmoded beliefs circulating in your mind. Due to being triggered into contraction, you protect and retract. To pacify your emotions, you reach for substances you know aren't good for you. The pattern is reinforced. And yet . . .

You've just been presented another chance to put your neuroplasticity to good use. You can use any and every minute opportunity to shift your awareness—and subsequently your biochemistry—into alignment with what you want to perceive and receive. Take a moment to practice with these simple instructions:

1. Feel the ground (earth) beneath you.

2. Feel the sky (heaven) above you.

3. Let your awareness pulsate between the two.

4. Notice as you do this that your insides feel expanded. You are giving your cells room to expand.

5. Notice as you do this that your mind—your awareness— feels bigger. You are giving your mind room to expand.

Now go back to what you were doing from this expanded mind-body perspective. Repeat a few times a day.

If the daily habits open gateways to a sacred, extraordinary life, easeful living is the crown jewel. It will arise as you gain traction with the other habits, and you can accelerate your shift with the tips below.

Your Bliss-Body

The Tantric yogis have long accessed easeful living via the bliss-body. Tantric teachings from the ninth- to eleventh-century writings emphasized the undulations of bliss emanating from our very nature. They drew attention to awakening the *anandamaya kosha*, the "sheath of bliss," that lies within us, closer to us than our body or our breath.

The Tantrikas emphasized that this is who we are, our inner nature, closer than our very flesh. They went to the moon and back writing about this realm. This intrinsic bliss field is within us all, surrounding the core of pure awareness or the ground of being. We can replenish and heal the wounds of unbridled separation consciousness with connection into the bliss sheath.

If you've never accessed the bliss-body teachings, chances are this sounds like cloud nine. Indeed, you may have a deep disconnect from both your bliss-body and from the backdrop of expanded awareness. The heart of intimacy issues—self-dislike issues, eating issues, addictions, anxiety, and depression—lies between the layers of self, all featuring a central disconnect with the bliss-body.

Even a repetitive mantra like "I don't like my thighs" speaks to the disconnect. When your awareness is seated in expanded consciousness, your baseline is love, respect, appreciation, gratitude. From this awareness you are also awake to the law of vibration—that nothing is in a static state. If you want to reshape your thighs, you reshape your thighs from a feeling of love and cooperation.

As you experience the gentle pleasantness that comes from the other nine habits, you're picking up the subtle, blissful sensations of the anandamaya kosha. As you deepen your habits and practices, you'll continue to home in on the center of the infinite—cracking the code of expanded awareness.

Certainty Anchors

When your day-to-day habits are simple and repetitive, you can enjoy amazing depth, connectedness, and success in other areas of your life. In his book *Uncertainty*, Jonathan Fields explains this phenomenon among highly creative people. He says throughout their day, highly creative people drop in certainty anchors—small repetitive rituals. The more creative you want to be, the more certainty anchors you want in your day that are centered around sitting in silence, food, sleep, exercise, work, shopping, and so forth. The more you live in simple rituals that work for your body, mind, and spirit, the more creative juice you free up. Your highly functional daily certainty anchors make you energy-efficient—freeing up space for clarity, for creativity, and for stepping toward potential.[4]

You can use certainty anchors with easeful living. I use the emotional trigger of stress for this habit. I've trained myself to zoom out to a bigger perspective when stress constricts my flow. Works like a charm.

Today Is a New Day

Unless you plant the seeds for tomorrow today, you shoot tomorrow in the foot. Most of us need more space. Our lives are busy and full. Our cups overflow, but not in an abundant kind of way. Our daily cups overflow in a turn-off-the-faucet-I'm-making-a-mess kind of way. When you align your day-to-day habits with even the smallest change, you experience both the energy and the peace that comes with the slightest increase of spaciousness.

Tomorrow ≠ a new day

Today = a new day

Time is intricately linked to space. When you don't have space, you feel like you don't have enough time. Time arises within space, so when you don't have time, it's really a space issue. If you open up space in your mind and in your body, you'll open up time in your life. If easeful living is inaccessible, go back to Habit 1: Eat an Earlier, Lighter Dinner. Open the space in your evening—and open the space of your tomorrow.

TIPS FOR EASEFUL LIVING

- Acquiesce your attention toward the backdrop behind this moment. Train your attention to ease, depth, and space.

- Give preference to connection with and compassion for others.

- Gift yourself time to go about your day to avoid perpetuating tension and stress.

- Use the five simple instructions I gave you earlier (on page 200) a few times a day.

- Meditate.

- Use the "ah" breaths as needed, the way premenstrual women use dark chocolate for emotional relief.

- Use the lower section of your lungs to breathe your way through life. Lengthen your exhalation when under stress.

- Spend less time with annoying and stressed-out people.

- Spend more time with relaxed, happy people who are living their lives on purpose.

- If you're stressed about money, take action. Tackle your issues, get the financial education you need, or take a financial therapy course. When you find new ways of being useful, you won't have a problem with money.

- If you're stressed about time, take a time management course and meditate. Meditation opens your perception of time.

- If you're stressed about your living environment, use the Marie Kondo method of clearing your space.

- If you have a negative mindset around poor self-worth, focus on being useful or helpful. When others appreciate your usefulness or helpfulness, take that in fully. Relax into your better sense of self and what you are becoming.

- Read stories of enlightened, awake people. Notice their habits, their mindsets, their beliefs, and the universal laws they honor in their actions.

Part 3

Conclusion

There Is No End Game

Over the past ten weeks, if you followed a habit chapter per week, you have been on an odyssey of habit evolution. Chances are you now see good- and bad-habit triggers without even looking for them. This is a sign that you are waking up to the next level of designing the body, life, and schedule you want.

You passed through a *diksha*—a rite of passage. You are the hero on this journey, and you've been initiated. You have traversed the parts of your day, shining the light of awareness on what exactly you do, what you choose, and what you want to reverse-engineer for optimization and automation.

You've made changes—some tiny, some bigger. You're automating those changes in how your triggers bring about those microhabits on a daily basis. At this point, you're in process. Your best choice is to go around the 10 Habits of Body Thrive again. Start with Habit 1. You'll go deeper, and the process will be easier this time.

As you learn, you grow. Your limitations disintegrate in the shadows of the competencies gained through your new triggers, your small improvements, and your desire to keep evolving. You know how to help yourself. You also know how to help others who want to uplevel how they feel.

The 10 Habits of Body Thrive wake up your sacred anatomy and align you to your sacred life. These habits are an initiation into your sacred life. The habits work on your subtle channels, opening you up to the flow of consciousness. As you become more conscious, you become more interconnected. Your care expands, and your sense of self expands to the point where you realize that you are evolution in action. You realize that the only way evolution can show up is as you and everyone and everything else right now.

For those born and raised in a family culture that didn't engage in these habits, the path to automating these habits is arduous and fraught with the setbacks of resistance and regression. Regardless of where you started, diksha is diksha. Once you get through a passage—skillfully and with the know-how to get through again—you will know how to help others along. At that point, you've arrived at the next level.

The Next Level—Dharma Up

After Body Thrive, the next level is about dharma, or living on purpose. The essential Body Thrive Habits enable you to upgrade your energy integrity. When you're living in integrity, you become a manifestation of life itself, growing into higher configurations while reorganizing into an enhanced, upgraded constellation. At this point, you enter the level of living deeper into your dharma.

Dharma means "duty" and "purpose." As you learn how to optimize your body, build your energy integrity, and own your constitution, you will get tested by old distractions and past patterns that can suck you backward. You break through those patterns using tapas, using the small steps of kaizen, engaging abhyasa, and learning from karma.

When you break through those patterns, you pass the test. You enter another realm of reality and potentiality. From a scientific viewpoint, you pass into a more advanced meme of human development. You are able to build your prana, your tejas, and your body ojas simultaneously and altogether.

Pause.

Look back at your old life, your uninformed habits, your old cravings and proclivities, your old temperament and beliefs. Was the old you—your old body and mind—though younger chronologically, more aged in body, mind, or spirit? Have you challenged your beliefs on aging and disease?

You are no longer who you were when you started this book. Of course, you didn't follow it perfectly; it was just one sweep.

Yet, just like when you're sweeping a dirty garage, the first sweep creates the biggest pile of filth for removal. With each subsequent sweep, the piles are smaller, and the garage starts to sparkle. Keep passing through the Body Thrive Habits in ten-week segments. The habits build on each other. You, too, sparkle more with each pass.

Building Blocks for Extraordinary Thrive

When you watch a typical superhero movie, the storyline goes something like this: Your superhero starts out remarkably ordinary (think Cinderella, Luke Skywalker, Neo). Something devastating calls the hero into initiation. The hero learns to overcome obstacles. In doing so, the hero changes and awakens to an innate sense that the world should be different. She wants bigger change. The hero goes after it. Then, shockingly, the goal turns out to be much harder to attain than expected.

The superhero-to-be is dismayed. Dismayed and deterred. Next, an auspicious helping hand comes along—a teacher, a fairy godmother, a funny-looking Jedi master with sagacious ears, an otherworldly inspirational leader, a Body Thrive coach—and a bond is formed. Something is learned. There is more struggle and innocence lost. The superhero gains her power. She changes, and in her changing, the world evolves. She passed the diksha. And then? A new world is possible.

This is the nature of nailing the habits. The Body Thrive Habits are core competencies of extraordinary health. The laws of cause and effect become much more obvious once you understand them. You choose to pay attention to the laws of nature: the biorhythmic clock, the law of cause and effect, the law of polarity, the law of increase. In doing so, you have more energy, more time, more connectivity, more joy. You become more human, or human+. These powers you gain from nailing the core competencies with repeated practice are what the yogis call *siddhis*. Siddhis are superpowers available to humans who practice the path to an awake life.

Human+

The Body Thrive Habits seem so obvious, so basic, that you may wonder if your ancestors had these human+ experiences. My sense is that, except in rare cases, they did not. A life closer to the earth? That, they had. But a life of greater interconnectivity? I doubt it. If we look back, women's right to vote is just a hundred years old, and racial segregation ended a little more than fifty years ago in the United States. Our ancestors were in survival mode, and most did not have the luxury or access to the education or free time we have today.

One hundred years ago, very few people had time to develop themselves because of disease, war, strife, weather, and all sorts of abuse including racism, sexism, and imperialism. For many people, the basics of food, water, shelter, and protection consumed most of their time. They may have gone to bed early, awoken early, and eaten a seasonal plant-based diet with inevitable intermittent fasting, but very few had the access to information or social freedoms that enable us to live these habits today. Access to information is improving almost everywhere, yet more than twice the population of the United States lives without access to clean water.[1] As broadband, mobile interconnectivity, and social sharing rise, we can help people around the world thrive together by moving ideas and resources to the places most needed.

Through the Body Thrive Habits you generate deep, sustaining energy. This energy awakens the capacity and the desire to go beyond your current perceived potential. You enter the phase of development where you can become who you have not yet been before. You wake up to a calling, a strong desire to make something bigger happen with your energy.

As you live the Body Thrive Habits, your level or dimension of consciousness also expands. You can digest the tough stuff life serves up. You experience new degrees of integrity, and with this comes the desire to be a force for positive evolution.

As you generate a resilient body and mind by residing in the deep rhythms of nature as *your* nature, you will naturally raise and refine your own vibration. You will naturally intuit your own next purpose. You will sense what you should do and who you will need to become next to do that. You will desire your life to be in accordance with the deeper meaning you now perceive through your dynamic biorhythms, invigorated from your Body Thrive Habits.

You are more capable now. You are more capable of positive impact that goes well beyond your self and your own thrive. You will want to use your energy surplus to generate life-positive actions that happen on a bigger scale or with greater depth. You are a more expansive version of yourself. While it's not the easy road, it's the natural evolution of a thriving human being.

Notice your new deeper desires as you dial in your Body Thrive Habits. This is the path of your potential becoming real.

Put what you learn each day into action. Optimize your personal hygiene with the Body Thrive Habits, and step into living as evolution in action. Free of your outdated habits, you no longer get sucked back into the mindset and patterning that keeps you trapped in the relative, in the small you, in cycles of repeating your past at the expense of our collective future.

At this stage, you come to your practices with a whole other level of care, commitment, and concern beyond yourself: aware of the steps you took to awaken your body, your dharma, and your life, and wanting to help others connect the dots to a better experience.

At this stage, your practices and sacred habits enable you to show up fully alive to collaborate. The ideas, projects, and people in your daily life are exciting and impactful. Centered, rooted, expansive, and receptive, you are more capable than ever. Your dharma expands—you're working on projects and with people you'd never imagined. People will thank you for just being you. Thank you for doing the work.

Round and Round We Go

If you get stuck in a rut, grab a friend. Go through Body Thrive together in ten weeks. It gets easier every time. Believe me, I speak from experience.

KITCHEN SADHANA

Enlightening Your Kitchen

WHAT TO DO

Schedule two hours every week or biweekly to prepare
foods for the week and align your kitchen to feed your soul.

WHY YOU WANT TO DO IT

Every week or fortnight, as a practice, spend a special chunk of time in your kitchen—roughly two
hours—doing things that make it easier to prepare
foods quickly and more easily during the everyday kind
of days in between.

HOW TO START

Get out your calendar and mark off two hours during
the morning of a day off. Purge your kitchen of stuff
you don't use anymore, and clean your cupboards.

Kitchen Sadhana invites you to have a discipline, a practice, around
how you keep your kitchen, and how you use it to create your body
(and the other bodies you feed). I first learned of kitchen sadhana

from Maya Tiwari's groundbreaking book for Westerners, *Ayurveda: A Life of Balance*. While most of the kitchen sadhana Tiwari spells out in her magnum opus doesn't look anything like what I actually do in my kitchen sadhana, two decades later the concept sticks. Yet, having special time set aside each week or fortnight to update, overhaul, and co-create with plants, making them into foods, can indeed become a sacred practice. The goal is simple—make your kitchen functional and your foods intentional, aligning with who you want to become.

When the Priests Were the Cooks

Once upon a time, the priestly Brahmin caste prepared the food for the king and his family. The priests were the cooks, as well as the spiritual, ethical, and political advisors. The idea was to have the energy of awake mindfulness—of God, the divine, and enlightenment—infused into the food, coupled with the alchemy of preparing food with attention to season and constitution for the king's health. And so it can be in your kitchen. The energies you bring into your kitchen, from your ingredients to your attitude, give rise to the energies and attitudes you experience from what you eat.

Sadhana means "spiritual practice." Any practice, or something you do repetitively with the goal of connecting with the highest, is sadhana. For this reason, kitchen sadhana becomes a natural, effortless part of a life connected to dharma. If you spend a chunk of time in the kitchen twice a month, taking care of specific activities that make future meal preparation faster, you'll save a ton of time and eat better. These activities can include things like purging your cabinets, restocking your grains, beans, seeds, or spices, making batches of living foods (such as sauerkraut, green powder, granola). We can take these activities and turn them into sadhana, or a practice with a spirit-revitalizing goal.

"Sadhana is a means where bondage becomes liberation," says yoga historian N. N. Bhattacharyya.[1] If kitchen work sounds like bondage to you, it just may become a gateway. Yoga master B. K. S. Iyengar reminds us that sadhana has everything to do with practice and action:

Sadhana is a discipline undertaken in the pursuit of a goal. *Abhyasa* is repeated practice performed with observation and reflection. *Kriya*, or action, also implies perfect execution with study and investigation. Therefore, sadhana, abhyasa, and kriya all mean one and the same thing. A *sadhaka*, or practitioner, is one who skillfully applies . . . mind and intelligence in practice toward a spiritual goal.[2]

The consequences are drastic. Without kitchen sadhana, you fall into food ruts, messy cupboards, convenience foods, and a less interconnected body. This practice disciplines you to set up your food-body for the week. Kitchen sadhana can be as easy as taking a two-hour chunk of time to go through your cupboards to see what you've got, get out your recipe books or go to a recipe website, fill out your Weekly Meal Planner, and write your grocery list. Kitchen sadhana pays big dividends:

- You save time.

- You eat better.

- You save money.

- Your kitchen becomes seasonal.

- Your kitchen becomes more useful.

- You'll become more relaxed and easeful as you eradicate the stress from feeding yourself (and your family) well on a day-to-day basis.

- You become healthier because you're designing your body through your kitchen practices.

Two hours of kitchen sadhana every other week enables me to put together delicious, homemade, nutrient-dense meals in less than twenty minutes. This comes in super-useful if you are in the overscheduled, undernurtured category. Other signs that you need this habit may include some of the following: you're packing a few extra pounds, you need better nutrition, you're holding stress, you don't feel nurtured, you enter your kitchen famished and just grab something quick, you don't have healthy food at the ready, and your kitchen doesn't feel sacred or well used.

Preparing Food from Scratch in the Modern Age

When you make your own food, you get good at adjusting recipes for your body, and soon you're cooking from scratch without recipes at all. You crave your own food. Eating out for more than a few consecutive meals or eating prepared foods lessens your power. Your mind isn't as clear. Your body isn't as strong. Your home isn't as nurturing. Why? Because your senses, hands, and intuition are attuned to what you need and subtly energize your staples.

Historically, humans selected and prepared their own food within family systems. If you're the household cook, you know how everyone else in the household likes their food. You know who likes cardamom more than cinnamon, who uses more salt or pepper, who needs more greens than grains. When your kitchen syncs with the seasons, climate, and plants that grow in your hood, you enter a deeper level of flow and ease.

Kitchen sadhana demands that you not only *own* your kitchen but that you revitalize the space biweekly. You get a spell of time to align how you feed yourself with how you want to be. Do you want to be lighter? Heavier? Warmer? Cooler? More nourished? Clearer? More cozy? You take these *gunas*, these attributes, and realign your food stores and kitchen atmosphere to feed your body with more accuracy. You can employ your living space, including your kitchen, to take on a dharma. Ask yourself:

- How can I use my home to serve my evolving habits?

- How can I organize it so it serves my goals?

- How can I use this space in the future to serve my evolving habits?

Think of everything you own—everything that takes up your space—as paying you rent. What is earning its keep by serving your needs? What takes up space, giving nothing in return? Be ruthless in your evaluation. The purpose of my kitchen is to nourish my body efficiently and with love. My kitchen evolves with me.

Without kitchen sadhana, foods sneak onto your shelves that aren't in alignment with who you want to become. Purge and pass on. The point is to ask yourself what needs to happen in your kitchen for the space to better serve your collective needs and help you align your diet with your goals—and then take action.

Start with a Purge

The very first kitchen sadhana session is a purge. Invite Buddhi, the enlightened version of yourself, to the party. Buddhi is your higher self—the part that has two-way communication between the self and the whole. The part that loves meditation and "gets" the concept of easeful living. Buddhi demands connection to being, and you know that requires clear space—sukha. Your Buddhi can make sukha happen in your kitchen with about twenty minutes and two cardboard boxes. Let your Buddhi scour your kitchen. One box is for stuff to give away to someone in need or the thrift store. The other is stuff you might want later, but you're not interested in now.

The key here is that you have to let your higher mind do the work. Your outdated patterns will try to sabotage you, coming up with powerful reasons to hold onto the box of graham crackers or kitchen tools you've never used. Remember, this is sadhana—a discipline. Buddhi gets face time and calls the shots. Here is an example from a Yogidetoxer named Jackie:

> Last weekend I took your declutter directions to heart
> and cleaned out my space. I have continued to get rid of
> so much stuff in my apartment. My home feels different.
> I am feeling lighter.

Buddhi knows what goes where. You're done with this. You'll need this later. When the two boxes are full, tape them shut. Label them "food and kitchen items for the thrift store" and "stuff I will review and give away in six months." Put the latter in your garage, put the former in your car.

Nice work. You created some sukha that enables the natural flow of ease. You'll be inspired to keep going. Finish your session by making a list of the activities that you'll do in two weeks during kitchen sadhana. This is a practice. Schedule it, and make it a recurring bimonthly event. It's not a one-shot deal. You're deepening your connection with the spirit of the kitchen—the spirit of food preparation. This is how your food and your body become sacred.

Batch-Tasking with Buddhi

Once your kitchen is clear and highly functional, you'll want to use your kitchen-sadhana task list to batch-task food preparation. There are two ways to look at kitchen sadhana:

1. Kitchen tasks

2. Homemade staples

Kitchen tasks are the realm of cleaning, organizing, and stocking. Check off the kitchen tasks you need to do.

- Clean the kitchen drawers and cupboards
- Fill in your Weekly Meal Planner
- Make a grocery list
- Clean the fridge (recruit help)
- Restock your kitchen staples
- Purge and restock your kitchen for the current season
- Refresh your spices (every six to twelve months)
- Harvest your garden
- Install a compost bin
- Turn the compost

Homemade staples are foods you only need to make once a week (like salad dressing), once a month (like granola), or once a year (like miso). Here are the staples I make, in order from weekly to annually.

- Salad dressings and sauces
- Roasted vegetables
- Boiled vegetables (in salty water)
- Soaked chia for porridge (keeps in fridge for a week)
- Stock for soups and other dishes
- Sprouted nuts and seeds
- Cookies or raw chocolate balls
- Hummus or bean dips
- Granola
- Raw crackers
- Pickled vegetables or sauerkraut
- Fruit rollups for the kid
- Green powders and superfood blends
- Herbal teas
- Miso paste

My Kitchen Sadhana in Action

I prefer to time-block my kitchen-sadhana tasks. I recommend starting with a Weekly Meal Planner (print a few from the *Body Thrive Workbook*). See what you can do in a time block to set yourself up for the week ahead. As you develop a rhythm with your food body, you will find that when and what you do in a kitchen sadhana session develops its own ease, rhythm, and efficiency. I'll unpack how I use my kitchen time efficiently and eat exceptionally well to share my process, but yours will likely be different. I prefer weekends; you may prefer another time. Like all habits, get in a groove and stick to it until you find a better habit. I keep a fridge list of what is next on my kitchen sadhana of the week. The list has specific to-dos. Here is an example for one session:

- Roast vegetables
- Boil vegetables

- Make lemon miso salad dressing
- Check miso in basement
- Harvest basil
- Make pesto
- Wash compost bin

Here is an example for another session I had recently:

- Make buckwheat granola
- Make honey-mustard vinaigrette
- Harvest two weeks of carrots
- Put the weeds in the dehydrator
- Pick chokecherries and rose hips

I like to have cooked vegetables around for making a soup or salad in a few minutes. Often, I walk in hungry for lunch or dinner and want to whip up a vegetable-based meal. I'll roast sweet potatoes, potatoes, beets, and sometimes cauliflower, onions, broccoli, or asparagus. The roots I'll throw in the oven whole. The others I'll toss with olive oil, salt, and pepper. The oven is hot, around 425 degrees. I'll turn on the oven and put a pot of salty water on the stove at the same time. The prep on this part is ten minutes max. The payoff for the next few days saves time and stress and leads to better meals.

I've found that many living foods, which are high in enzymes and great for optimal digestion, absorption, and elimination, are easier to prepare in batches and stay fresh. Sauerkraut, sprouted buckwheat granola, soaked chia, and homemade dried green powders are staples I use sometimes daily. Making staples in batches saves tons of time in the kitchen and makes meal prep fast. Living foods are packed with enzymes, nutrients, and prana. Enzymes and prana decrease with leftovers and traditional canning methods. With fermenting and dehydrating, enzymes and prana remain intact. This is wicked cool.

Raw buckwheat granola is one of my breakfast staples, as I prefer to start the day raw. First, I have a wild or domesticated green smoothie. After that is digested (twenty minutes) I often move on to chia porridge with a handful of buckwheat granola on top. Like many raw foods, buckwheat granola doesn't take much hands-on time to prepare a month's supply, but it does require a variety of very quick steps spread out over time.

When "make buckwheat granola" is on my kitchen-sadhana list, that weekend I start a few days ahead of the session with one-minute tasks. A few days before, I'll soak my buckwheat in a big bowl of water. This takes about one minute to do, then it sits overnight. In the morning I drain the buckwheat and spread it on a big cookie sheet. I cover it with a light dishtowel and find unused counter space in my kitchen to let the buckwheat babies grow. Every morning and night for a day or two, I will lift the towel and very gently fluff the buckwheat babies. I don't rinse. Just fluff. When I'm in Mexico, it's humid and mold grows, so I rinse and fluff twice a day, and they sprout in half the time. The night before my kitchen-sadhana session, I'll soak my raisins and dates in one bowl and my almonds in another. So far, I've invested about five minutes of time total.

On kitchen-sadhana day, I'm ready. On the list is to make buckwheat granola and honey-mustard vinaigrette, harvest the carrots, and pick rose hips and chokecherries for wild tea. I'll start with the granola. The time to combine the ingredients in the blender and spread it on dehydrator trays and clean up is ten to fifteen minutes. Now I have enough homemade granola for a month. I make a salad vinaigrette (five minutes) and harvest and wash the carrots (forty minutes). I have almost an hour to take my kid for a walk in the woods to pick the rose hips and chokecherries. These grow in absurd abundance, and I know my patches. No sweat.

This is the nature of kitchen sadhana. Once you have your routines dialed in, you access long-term benefits. You save buckets of time, connect your body to your food, maybe even to your ecosystem, and eat higher quality nutrients for less money.

If you want to prepare the most nurturing nutrition for your body, is there a way to make it more organized, efficient, sacred, or enjoyable? Take a moment and write a list of ideas. Invite the sadhana aspect into the practice. You'll love how putting in some enlightened elbow grease once a week will enable you to waltz into your kitchen for great, quick-prep meals every day. You'll be more relaxed and aware of what your body wants.

As my friend chef Johnny Brannigan taught me, "The consciousness of the chef is the most important ingredient in the food." You get to become both the priest and the king.

List of Worksheets

Download your free copy of the *Body Thrive Workbook* at bodythrive.com/free. It contains these worksheets, which correspond to the 10 Body Thrive Habits.

Worksheet Title	Corresponding Chapter/Habit
Your What, Your Why & Your Anchor	Crash Course on Habit Evolution
Better Habits Monthly Chart	Any habit
Weekly Meal Planner	Habit 1: Eat an Earlier, Lighter Dinner
Food & Focus for Earlier, Lighter Dinners	Habit 1: Eat an Earlier, Lighter Dinner
What Time Is Dinner?	Habit 1: Eat an Earlier, Lighter Dinner
Early-to-Bed Flow Chart	Habit 2: Go to Bed Early
Golden Milk Recipe & Sleep Tonics	Habit 2: Go to Bed Early
Checklist to Start Your Day Right	Habit 3: Start Your Day Right
Dos & Don'ts for Start Your Day Right	Habit 3: Start Your Day Right

Worksheet Title	Corresponding Chapter/Habit
Guide to Start Your Day Right Mindful Breathing	Habit 3: Start Your Day Right
Intuition Worksheet for Start Your Day Right	Habit 3: Start Your Day Right
Breath-Body Programs Online	Habit 4: Bestir Your Breath-Body
Workout Chart	Habit 4: Bestir Your Breath-Body
Hard, Moderate & Easy Workouts	Habit 4: Bestir Your Breath-Body
Species I Eat List	Habit 5: Fuel Yourself with a Plant-Based Diet
20 Tips for a Plant-Based Diet	Habit 5: Fuel Yourself with a Plant-Based Diet
Food Journal	Habit 5: Fuel Yourself with a Plant-Based Diet
Self-Massage Recipes	Habit 6: Self-Massage Your Body
Dos & Don'ts for Self-Massage	Habit 6: Self-Massage Your Body
Oil & Orifices for Self-Massage	Habit 6: Self-Massage Your Body
Start Meditating Worksheet	Habit 7: Sit in Silence
Healthier Eating Simple Checklist	Habit 8: Heed the Healthier Eating Guidelines
Dos & Don'ts for Healthier Eating Guidelines	Habit 8: Heed the Healthier Eating Guidelines
Do I Have Ama?	Habit 8: Heed the Healthier Eating Guidelines
Ayurvedic Tongue Chart	Habit 9: Come to Your Senses
Blank Tongue Charts	Habit 9: Come to Your Senses
My Tongue Analysis Chart	Habit 9: Come to Your Senses
Eye Care Practices	Habit 9: Come to Your Senses
Nasal Care Practices	Habit 9: Come to Your Senses

Worksheet Title	Corresponding Chapter/Habit
Easeful Living Evaluation	Habit 10: Live in Ease
Evaluation Worksheet	Habit 10: Live in Ease
Choose Your Orientation Worksheet	Habit 10: Live in Ease
Sketch Your Emerging Orientation	Habit 10: Live in Ease
Trading Bad for Better Worksheet 1	Any habit
Trading Bad for Better Worksheet 2	Any habit
Identity-Evolving Worksheet	Any habit
Keystone Habit Worksheet	Any habit
Peer Support Worksheet	Any habit
Payoff Worksheet	Any habit
You & Resistance	Any habit
Low or High Motivation Worksheet	Any habit
Limiting Beliefs/Higher Truths	Any habit
Core Strategies to Change Habits	Any habit

Create a Book Club for *Body Thrive*

L ocal yoga studios, meditation centers, student health classes, and holistic wellness practices can create a book group to integrate Body Thrive in community. The 10 Habits of Body Thrive naturally lend themselves to a ten-week format, and the best way for a book club to dive into the book and workbook is over a ten-week period.

Below are some suggested questions to help start off and guide the discussion each week. If you follow along with this format, your group will have to read and discuss the first few opening chapters along with Habit 1 and the two closing chapters with Habit 10. Or, you could bypass those chapters and concentrate solely on the habits. Whatever works best for you and your peeps. Be sure to use A Crash Course on Habit Evolution on page 19 as a foundation as you work through the book, consulting it as a reference over the course of the ten weeks. Use the strategies in this chapter to troubleshoot any difficulties working through the habits.

The online *Body Thrive Workbook* accompanies the book, which is free to everyone in your group; you'll find it at bodythrive.com/free. Tell your group members to print the workbook, put it in a binder, and bring it to your meetings!

Discuss *Body Thrive* with Your Home Book Club

If you have an existing book club that reads a book a month, you'll need to decide as a group if you want to read this book over ten weeks, or stick with the standard format. I recommend reading it over ten weeks so your group has time to dive into and implement each of the habits. If you want to go the book-a-month route, after you've read and discussed *Body Thrive*, you might choose a book for the following month that has a wellness, spiritual, or inspirational message. I suggest: *Better Than Before* by Gretchen Rubin, *The Surrender Experiment* by Michael Singer, *Choose Yourself* by James Altucher, *The Life-Changing Magic of Tidying Up* by Marie Kondo, or *Wild Edibles* by Sergei Boutenko. Any of these will complement and work well with the 10 Habits of Body Thrive.

Create a Virtual Book Club for *Body Thrive*

Don't discount the power and possibility of creating a book club in a virtual community. Maybe everyone who's interested in a book club has a crazy schedule, and finding time to meet up in person is like trying to herd cats. Or maybe your friends and family are sprinkled all over the country, or all over the world. You can still create a space for meaningful discussions and provide each other with support as you work through the Body Thrive Habits via social networks like Google+ and Facebook.

Book Club Questions

How Are You Designing Your Body?
Q: On a scale of 1 to 10, what is your level of commitment to *doing* this book together for the next ten weeks? Simply be honest with yourself and others.

How to Have a Body According to Ayurveda
Q: What struck you personally about the three causes of disease according to Ayurveda?
Q: How is "not learning from your past" playing out in your choices right now? Do you have habits that you'd like to shift? If so, what are they?

A Crash Course on Habit Evolution

Q: What do you want right now in your lifestyle? Time? Energy? Sleep? Better food? Better daily flow? Get clear on your "what" and share.

Q: Why do you want that right now? (Example: I want more sleep each night so that I can feel great every day.)

Q: Which of the habit-change strategies is most appealing to you? (Example: group support, kaizen, anchor statements, etc.)

Habit 1: Eat an Earlier, Lighter Dinner

Q: How can you apply kaizen, or a 1 percent improvement, to eating earlier or lighter this week?

Q: What time do you want to commit to eating dinner this week (five to seven nights)?

Q: How can you use one of the techniques from A Crash Course on Habit Evolution to make a plan that fits what you want to do, and is doable?

Habit 2: Go to Bed Early

Q: Who here has a body that needs more sleep? How much more?

Q: What time do you want to commit to going to bed this week (five to seven nights)?

Q: How can you reverse-engineer your new habit?

Q: What do you want to add or take away from your evening routine?

Q: Which exercises from the workbook have you found most helpful?

Habit 3: Start Your Day Right

Q: What are the biggest obstacles keeping you from becoming an early riser? Can you identify any limiting beliefs in those obstacles?

Q: How many of us wake up, hydrate, and poop every morning?

Q: What practice helps you open to a bigger perspective first thing? Gratitude? Prayer? Meditation? Journaling? If you don't have a practice, which one-minute practice do you want to try this week?

Habit 4 : Bestir Your Breath-Body

Q: How many of us actually move first thing in the morning?

Q: What would have to change for you to accommodate a twenty-minute breath-body practice as part of an every morning routine?

Q: Can you create a Fogg statement to help establish this routine? Right after I _____, I will (insert whatever movement appeals to you).

Q: Does the tracking worksheet help you plan your workouts and stay on track? (See the free, online workbook.)

Habit 5: Fuel Yourself with a Plant-Based Diet

Q: How diverse is your current diet? How many plant species did you eat this past week?

Q: How is your mindset regarding diet changing as you become more aware of plant species, plant parts, and seasonal eating?

Q: What new plant species can you add to your diet this week? This season?

Q: What is a "yes, and" statement you could use to eat a more nutrient-diverse, seasonal, local diet? Such as, "Yes, I eat a healthy diet, and this week I'm going to hunt for a vegetable at the market that I don't know how to cook."

Interlude: How to Evolve Your Habits in Relationships

Q: As you journey through *Body Thrive*, who are your Uplifters/Champions/Upholders?

Q: Who are the Middlers? The Backsliders?

Q: How can you navigate your relationships to support your evolution?

Q: Where can you find the supportive relationships you are missing?

Habit 6: Self-Massage Your Body

Q: Do you currently have a self-massage practice with oil, lotion, or dry-brushing? What did you learn from this chapter?

Q: Can you create an anchor statement to use with self-massage to become an even better caretaker of your body?

Q: Do you know what is in the substances you put on your skin with moisturizers, sunscreen, or makeup? If not, are you going to look it up on the Environmental Working Group website (ewg.org)?

Q: Can you alter your morning routine to include self-massage with dry-brushing or oil three times a week? What trigger will you use to automate this habit?

Habit 7: Sit in Silence

Q: Do you want to start meditating or up the ante on your current practice? If so, why? And what might change, evolve, or deepen in your life?

Q: What are the biggest obstacles keeping you from a daily meditation practice?

Q: What practices appeal to you the most? Which ones will have the biggest long-term impact?

Q: How much time can you consistently commit to your meditation practice at this phase in your life, without fail? Apply kaizen!

Q: If you have an existing practice, what could make it more effective?

Habit 8: Heed the Healthier Eating Guidelines

Q: Which of the Healthier Eating Guidelines are you incorporating into your habits?

Q: How often do you eat during the day? Do you snack between meals?

Q: How many of the six tastes are you currently eating?

Q: What are your outdated patterns in relation to the Healthier Eating Guidelines? Do you have beliefs you are ready to challenge?

Habit 9: Come to Your Senses

Q: How does *asatmendriyartha samyoga* show up in your life? How are you misusing your senses?

Q: What organ-care routine can you slip into your morning schedule? Tongue scraping? Oil pulling? Eye palming? Lubing the nose and ears?

Q: Which of the habits from earlier in the course are becoming automatic for you?

Q: What habit-evolution techniques from A Crash Course on Habit Evolution are you finding most effective as you incorporate the Body Thrive Habits?

Habit 10: Live in Ease
Q: How do you orient yourself in your day—through stress or ease? Are you noticing that you have a choice?
Q: Can you build triggers into your day to pause and recognize if you are in ease or in stress?
Q: How do the prior Body Thrive Habits align you with space and time? Do you feel more spaciousness in your day-to-day? Do you have more time? More intrinsic joy?
Q: Is there someone whose easeful, enlightened existence is an inspiration for you? Can you "fake it until you make it" to cultivate ease in your life this week?

There Is No End Game
Q: Revisit your "why" and your "what" from the book club questions for A Crash Course on Habit Evolution. What is changing in your life due to your ten-week Body Thrive journey? How is your day—and your life—different?
Q: Do you feel a momentum to your progress? Do you feel half-baked—like you're not quite done with this yet? Do you want to start again with Habit 1 and go deeper into Body Thrive?
Q: How have these habits challenged you to grow and change?
Q: What habit is your keystone habit? What habits do you need to work on?

Kitchen Sadhana: Enlightening Your Kitchen
Q: Were you inspired to purge and update your kitchen into alignment with your Body Thrive Habits?
Q: What simple steps can you take to prepare your food earlier in the week or earlier in the day?
Q: When will you schedule time in your week to batch-task and simplify your food preparation for the next spell?
Q: What will you do during your next kitchen-sadhana session?

Overarching Questions

Q: What part of the book resonated with you the most?

Q: Which habit is your keystone habit? (It's the one that clicks the other habits into place.)

Q: How has your journey through *Body Thrive* impacted your body, your mind, your spirit, and/or your relationships?

Q: Which worksheets from the free workbook have you found most helpful?

Q: If you love how you feel, do you want to coach others through the process? If so, go to bodythrive.com/coach.

Inspiration from Body Thrive
Course Members

R ead the breakthrough stories from members who invested in live Body Thrive coaching with Cate and the community for one year:

"Doing Body Thrive has brought me back to myself, back to home."

CAROLYN BOND

"It is absolutely insane to me what a massive impact small shifts in my daily routine have made." **FRANNIE FERRARA**

"Living the 10 Habits of Body Thrive not only changed my life dramatically at the get-go, but there is a nonstop, continuous evolution occurring. I am becoming a new person every day. I'm creating the me I want to be and the life I want to live!" **DR. BETH CLAXTON, OB-GYN**

"Body Thrive has changed me as a person. After feeling overwhelmed, fat, and bloated, I am now in tune with my body, mind, and spirit. Changing the habits of a fifty-eight-year-old was easy when guided by Cate Stillman the easy, practical way. They are no longer habits of change but habits that are truly part of my everyday being." **BATOOL MERALI**

"Body Thrive is more than a ten-week crash course on how to feel better. It challenges me to listen to my intuition and let it guide me in all aspects of my life. I am learning to look at life as a dynamic experience, one in which I have a central role in creating every single moment." HEATHER FERRILL

"Body Thrive is giving me what I need the most in this crucial and stormy time of my life: the ability to recognize my needs and my voice, and a wonderful community to belong to!" M. MAR DÍAZ HERRERO

"I loved this program—I have so much more to do to learn and grow within myself. I feel better; I have a better insight into the food I put into my body and where I am in my daily routine. My energy and mental state are much clearer, and I have better habits to keep attending to. I think I would like to do it again to ingrain the habits even more. Body Thrive is amazing. Thank you." WENDI BUICK

"We live in Nature's house. She freely offers her playground for us to enjoy. The least we can do for this blessing is to align with Her and follow Her lead. Body Thrive guides us on this path of deeper commitment to ourselves and the world around us. Accepting Body Thrive's invitation is affirming life and stepping up to say "yes" to a bigger possibility. This is a game changer! I'm so glad I'm all in! Thank you, Cate!" JAMIE TURNER ALLISON

"Body Thrive taught me how to eat right for my body, and I lost ten pounds without even trying." VANESSA SULZER

"Before Body Thrive, my life was filled with the "dos and don'ts" of living a healthy lifestyle, which is always changing based on the current research, studies, or fads. After integrating the Body Thrive Habits into my life, I let go of those dos and don'ts for good. I now feel more tuned in to my body than I ever have before. I'm also watching my clients evolve into healthier individuals with the same confidence and ease as they tune in to their bodies too!" SHELLY AARON

"I was on the path before I began Body Thrive, but the practices have deepened, and they have more traction now. What I'm grateful for is the subtle identity shift from being one with good intentions to one who can pull them off. Thank you, Cate and Company, for putting together this ingenious package of mind-blowing material, inspiration, and wholehearted community support!" JUDY ORLOFF

"Experiencing Body Thrive as both a student and a coach was truly empowering. To work on and be witness to very personal transformations in a supportive, community-oriented environment brought a whole new level of ownership and self-love to my experience of embodied living. I'll always be grateful for this community." DINA CROSTA

"I have made peace with my body, and I'm working with my natural rhythms instead of fighting them. It feels not only okay, but wonderful, to inhabit myself. The visible and palpable changes (more calm, less weight!) on the surface hint at a true sea change that is going on underneath. Each habit paves the way for the next one, so that I find myself experimenting with new habits that I never thought I would, and I'm finding them more supportive and nourishing than I could have imagined. Very grateful."

JENNY FAULKNER CAMPBELL

"Since beginning Body Thrive five weeks ago, I have lost eight pounds! No dieting, no counting carbs or calories, just following the program as much as I can. Thanks Cate Stillman!" MICHELE SUMMERS COLÓN

"Body Thrive—indeed! I have more energy; a more loving, kind relationship with myself; and a cleaner diet—and my self-integrity has deepened. I have a community of peeps who are heading down the same path. As both a student and a coach, I am deeply grateful to be part of this tribe. It's amazing! I'm in my second round of Body Thrive right now and can feel the process continuing to fine-tune my daily rhythms. Body Thrive is a simple, straightforward approach with a deeply profound outcome."

JAMIE LYNN WORSTER

"Body Thrive means connection, access, and acceptance for me. I'm connecting on a deeper level to my body, my mind, my nature, and my ability to access and apply the wisdom of Ayurveda in my life on a daily basis. Finally, with Cate's emphasis on the science of habits, I now accept that I can slowly work through adopting these habits and make them my own. I'm so grateful for all the support, content, and Cate's amazing ability to be a catalyst for growth and change on many levels. You rock, Cate!"   TRACY GRAVES

Yogahealer Resources

Listen to Cate on her *Yogahealer Podcast*

Free Yogidetox recipe ebook at Yogidetox.com/free

Want to coach the Body Thrive Habits? Start your introductory free training: bodythrive.com/coach

For pregnancy and postpartum Body Thrive tips, get Cate's free ebook: mamabirthing.com

Free Ayurveda training with Cate: yogahealer.com/ayurveda

Glossary

A

abhyanga is the practice of daily massage from Ayurveda.

abhyasa is an intentional, repetitive practice done for spiritual evolution or long-term gain.

adhikara means "studentship" and implies building authority or ownership on a subject.

agni is the biological fire or ignition that governs metabolism, including digestion, absorption, and assimilation. As the power of heat and light in the subtle body, agni gives rise to willpower, wisdom, and insight.

ahamkara is the ego or the experience of identifying ourselves as separate and limited, enabling the soul to experience individualism.

ama means "uncooked" or "undigested," referring to anything that exists in a state of incomplete transformation. Physically, it refers to food that hasn't been digested properly. Mentally and emotionally, it refers to impressions that haven't been fully processed.

ananda is the bliss that arises from our inner nature.

anandamaya kosha is the subtlest sheath, the innermost layer of the self, which connects our infinite self to our intuition. Its energetic vibration is ananda—the highest truth, beauty, and bliss.

apana vayu is the downward flow of prana and is responsible for bowel function.

asatmendriyartha samyoga is a cause of disease due to using our senses (sight, hearing, taste, touch, smell) inappropriately.

atman refers to the infinite self—the spirit, which is unchanging, eternal, and conscious—distinct from both the mind and physical body.

B

brahmamuhurta is the time of the god Brahma, referring to *muhurta*, the time before sunrise—the most auspicious time for meditation, expanded awareness, gaining knowledge, or breaking patterns.

buddhi is our higher intelligence, which has access to expanded awareness on one hand and the data from our lived experience on the other.

C

chakra is one of the human body's seven subtle-energy centers (or wheels or vortexes) where matter and consciousness meet along the spine, from tailbone to crown.

charya refers to the potential to align our habits with the laws and rhythms of nature for optimal health.

D

dharma is our duty to society and the greater purpose of our life.

diksha is a rite of passage that allows us to transcend our current limitations.

dinacharya is the daily habits or routines that are essential for evolutionary wellness, expanded consciousness, and optimal physical, mental, and emotional health.

dosha refers to the three energies that create the constitution of everything living: anabolism (kapha), metabolism (pitta) and catabolism (vata).

dukha literally translates to "dirty space," and implies suffering.

E

ekagrata is the one-pointed focus that arises from focus as a
discipline to experience undisturbed attention.

K

kaizen is the relentless improvement toward perfection, based on
active learning, rigorous practice, and healthy skepticism. In
Japanese, *kai* means "change," and *zen* means "ideal state."

kapha means "to flourish by water." It's one of the triadic forces or doshas
(along with pitta and vata). Kapha generates cohesion or holding
cells together, protection, and repair. Kapha qualities are heavy, slow,
steady, solid, cold, soft, and oily.

karma is the law of cause and effect.

karna purana is an ear therapy in which oil is held in the ears for
a few moments. This lubricates the delicate filaments of the ear
canal, which sharpens hearing and removes impurities.

kitchari is a one-pot comfort food dish of rice, split mung-beans,
and curried spices sautéed in ghee. It can both detoxify and
rejuvenate.

koshas are the five layers of the self: the physical body, energy body,
mind body, intelligence body, and bliss-body. The five layers
emanate from and are saturated by our infinite nature, moving us
from gross to subtle, or obvious to elusive.

krama refers to chronology, or a special sequence in time, used to
create a desired effect.

kula is a community of the heart, or a dedicated spiritual community.

M

maha vaha srota is the mouth-to-anus channel of the digestive tract,
the fundamental channel of our physical body.

mahavakya means to use the power of the word to anchor your
awareness in the greatest capacity of yourself.

marma is an energetic intersection between the subtle and physical
bodies, similar to an acupressure point.

muhurta is the early morning hours before sunrise.

N

nadi is a channel or stream that carries consciousness and energy from the subtle body to the physical body.

nasya is the therapy of snorting therapeutic oil into the nostrils to open the breathing passages, shift the mental/emotional state, or relieve conditions such as allergies, sinusitis, headaches, or colds.

netra basti is an Ayurvedic therapy that bathes the eyes in ghee to restore tired eyes.

nimesha is the contracting energy of *spanda*, akin to closing one's eyes. It is the experience of closing one's eyes, folding inward, closing down, rooting. It is the opposite of *unmesha*, the movement of expansion.

O

ojas is our deep, vital energy reserve, which sustains physical and psychological stability and endurance and enables immunity, endurance, calm, and contentment. It is the fuel for health and growth.

P

panchakarma refers to the five actions that are done in a traditional Ayurvedic detoxification process.

parinama is being out of harmony with the daily, monthly (menstrual), seasonal, and/or time-of-life rhythms and cycles of nature.

pitta is one of the triadic forces or doshas (along with kapha and vata). Pitta controls digestion, metabolism, and energy production. The primary function of pitta is transformation. The qualities of pitta are hot, light, intense, penetrating, pungent, sharp, and acidic.

prajnaparadha is a cause of disease that occurs when we violate or don't embody what we've learned from our past. *Prajna* is direct insight into the truth. *Aparadha* means to violate or offend our own insight. Put together, it's when we transgress against that which we know to be true.

prana is the life-giving force of the breath, which coordinates our breath, senses, and mind, allowing us to become aware, flexible, adaptable, and growth oriented. It is the subtle energy of data behind all mind-body functions, and the catalyst for manifestation and evolution.

pranayama is a yogic conscious breathing practice designed to optimize one's vital energy.

purna means "fullness" or "completeness." Also known as *purnina*.

purnatva is the perfection that is the essence of all things.

R

raja means "king," "prince," or "ruler."

rajas is one of the triadic qualities of nature (the other two being sattva and tamas) and associated with energetic movement and passion.

ritucharya is seasonal housekeeping of your body-mind—the removal of the seasonal buildup of ama, which helps create space for decelerated, graceful aging.

S

sadhaka is one who is devoted to truth.

sadhana means a practice or discipline that leads to an aligned life.

sama agni is when digestion is healthy.

samskara is a recycled or stuck behavioral or thought pattern as a result of perpetuating tendencies in the subconscious mind.

sangha is a spiritual community, like a *kula* but more broad.

sankalpa is an intention formed by the heart and mind to direct attention and refine the deeper reason behind the intention.

sattva or **sattvic** refers to one of the triadic qualities of nature (the other two being rajas and tamas) that arises from aligned action and that generates light, peace, and interconnectivity.

Savasana is Corpse Pose, traditionally done at the end of yoga or pranayama practice to induce a deep, subtle integration of the preceding practice.

shakti is the female principle of divine energy moving and manifesting the universe.

shri is the spark of divinity.

siddhis are abilities that arise from yogic practices.

sneha means both "oil" and "love."

spanda is the universal principle of vibration connected to the law of polarity—the pulsations between expansion and contraction with everything and everyone. Unmesha and nimesha together are spanda.

subtle body is made up of impressions received from our five senses (hearing, touch, sight, taste, and smell), which generate our energetic qualities, emotions, senses, and intelligence.

sukha literally means "clean space" and implies the ease that arises from aligned action.

sushumna nadi is the main energetic channel of the subtle anatomy, which runs the north/south axis of the nervous system from crown to root.

svastha means "seated in oneself" or "integrated in body, mind, and spirit." Svastha is the basis of health in Ayurveda.

svatantriya describes our inner nature as completely free.

T

tamas is one of the triadic qualities of nature (the other two being sattva and rajas) and manifests as inertia, motionlessness, and resistance, creating obstacles and obstructions to counteract the movement of rajas.

tapas is the rub or heat that is generated by disciplined action. Tapas renders light.

tejas is our inner radiance, derived from the subtle energy of fire and the positive essence of pitta dosha. Tejas fires up our drive and aspirations to evolve.

U

unmesha is the expanding component of spanda, akin to opening one's eyes. It is the experience of unfolding, opening, blossoming. It is the opposite of nimesha, or the movement of contraction.

V

vaidya is an Ayurvedic doctor who is versed in the Vedas (Hindu scriptures).

vata is one of the triadic forces or doshas (along with kapha and pitta). Vata governs movement in the body, including breathing, circulation, digestion, elimination, and nervous activity. It moves the other doshas. Its qualities are cold, light, dry, irregular, rough, moving, quick, and changeable.

vinayam combines training, discipline, and cultured mannerism (from training) with humbleness. Vinayam occurs when we are humble to our higher truth and disciplined about training our habits and mannerisms around that which we know to be better.

viveka means discrimination, or the action or ability to distinguish or perceive differences. It is the power to differentiate between right and wrong, real and apparent, eternal and transient, better and worse.

Y

yoga is the practice of uniting the separate self into the perspective of wholeness.

yogis are people who practice yoga and the art of yoking together their personal mind, body, and spirit into optimal health and higher awareness for planetary interconnectivity and the good of all.

Notes

How to Have a Body According to Ayurveda
1. William Durant, *The Story of Philosophy: The Lives and Opinions of the World's Greatest Philosophers*, 1st ed. (New York: Simon and Schuster, 1926).
2. Sadhguru, "The Significance of 108—Why Is It So Important?" December 29, 2014, Isha Foundation, isha.sadhguru.org/us /en/wisdom/article/the-significance-of-108.

A Crash Course on Habit Evolution
1. James Clear, "How Willpower Works: The Science of Decision Fatigue and How to Avoid Bad Decisions," accessed October 1, 2018, lifehack.org/317884/how-willpower-works-the-science -decision-fatigue-and-how-avoid-bad-decisions.
2. William James, *The Principles of Psychology: Volume I* (New York: Henry Holt and Company, 1890), psychclassics.yorku .ca/James/Principles.
3. B. J. Fogg, "3 Steps to Changing Behavior," accessed October 1, 2018, foggmethod.com.
4. Charles Duhigg, "How Habits Work," accessed October 1, 2018, charlesduhigg.com/how-habits-work.
5. Chris Winfield, "This Is Warren Buffett's Best Investment Advice," *Time*, July 23, 2015, time.com/3968806 /warren-buffett-investment-advice.

Habit 1: Eat an Earlier, Lighter Dinner
1. "Body Measurements," Centers for Disease Control and Prevention's National Center for Health Statistics, May 3, 2017, cdc.gov/nchs/fastats/body-measurements.htm.

2. "Prevalence of Obesity among Adults and Youth: United States, 2015–2016," Centers for Disease Control and Prevention, October 2017, cdc.gov/nchs/data/databriefs/db288.pdf.

3. Remy C. Martin-Du Pan et al., "The Role of Body Position and Gravity in the Symptoms and Treatment of Various Medical Diseases," *Swiss Medical Weekly* 134, nos. 37–38 (September 18, 2004): 543–551, doi.org/10.4414/smw.2004.09765.

4. Micah Abraham, "Anxiety Always Comes with Shallow Breathing," Calm Clinic, last updated September 28, 2017, calmclinic.com/anxiety/symptoms/shallow-breathing.

5. Akash K. Agrawal, C. R. Yadav, and M. S. Meena, "Physiological Aspects of Agni," *An International Quarterly Journal of Research in Ayurveda* 31, no.1 (July–September 2010): 395–398, doi.org/10.4103/0974-8520.77159.

6. Koert van Ittersum and Brian Wansink, "Plate Size and Color Suggestibility: The Delboeuf Illusion's Bias on Serving and Eating Behavior," *Journal of Consumer Research* 39, no. 2 (August 1, 2012): 215–228, doi.org/10.1086/662615.

Habit 2: Go to Bed Early

1. "Allergy Facts and Figures," Asthma and Allergy Foundation of America, accessed October 1, 2018, aafa.org/page/allergy-facts.aspx.

2. Julia Rodriguez, "CDC Declares Sleep Disorders Are a Public Health Epidemic," Advanced Sleep Medicine Services, accessed October 1, 2018, sleepdr.com/the-sleep-blog/cdc-declares-sleep-disorders-a-public-health-epidemic.

3. Yosef Brody, "Losing Sleep in the 21st Century," *Psychology Today*, May 7, 2013, psychologytoday.com/us/blog/limitless/201305/losing-sleep-in-the-21st-century.

4. Ann Pietrangelo and Stephanie Watson, "The Effects of Sleep Deprivation on Your Body," Healthline, June 5, 2017, healthline.com/health/sleep-deprivation/effects-on-body.

5. "Researchers Are Studying the Line Between Sleep and Cancer," Cancer Exercise Training Institute, April 10, 2018, thecancerspecialist.com/2018/04/10/researchers-are-studying-the-link-between-sleep-and-cancer.

6. Elizabeth Millard, "The Cortisol Curve," Experience Life, March 2016, experiencelife.com/article/the-cortisol-curve.

7. Eve Van Cauter et al., "The Impact of Sleep Deprivation on Hormones and Metabolism," *Medscape #7*, no.1 (2005), medscape.org/viewarticle/502825.

8. Van Cauter et al., "The Impact of Sleep Deprivation."

9. See note 2. Also "Drowsy Driving and Automobile Crashes: 1998 NCSDR/NHTSA Expert Panel on Driver Fatigue and Sleepiness," National Highway Traffic Safety Administration, US Department of Transportation, April 1998, nhtsa.gov /sites/nhtsa.dot.gov/files/808707.pdf.

10. Swami Lakshmanjoo, "The Theory of Letters That Expand the Universe and Quantum Reality," accessed October 1, 2018, inannareturns.com/articles/shivasutras/sutra002-07.htm.

11. W. Sayorwan et al., "The Effects of Lavender Oil Inhalation on Emotional States, Autonomic Nervous System, and Brain Electrical Activity," *Journal of the Medical Association of Thailand* 95, no. 4 (April 2012): 598–606.

12. "Night Owls May Be More Sedentary, Less Motivated to Exercise," American Academy of Sleep Medicine, June 3, 2014, aasm.org /night-owls-may-be-more-sedentary-less-motivated-to-exercise.

13. "'Night Owls' Drive Much Worse in the Morning," *ScienceDaily*, June 27, 2014, sciencedaily.com/releases /2014/06/140627094553.htm.

14. Jessica Rosenberg et al., "Early to Bed, Early to Rise: Diffusion Tensor Imaging Identifies Chronotype-Specificity," *NeuroImage* 84 (January 1, 2014): 428–434, doi.org/10.1016/j.neuroimage .2013.07.086.

15. Linda Geddes, "First Physical Evidence of Why You're an Owl or a Lark," *New Scientist*, September 30, 2013, newscientist.com/article /dn24292-first-physical-evidence-of-why-youre-an-owl-or-a-lark.

16. American Academy of Sleep Medicine, "Night Owls May Be More Sedentary, Less Motivated to Exercise"; University of Granada, "Night Owls Drive Much Worse in the Morning"; Jessica Rosenberg et al., "Early to Bed, Early to Rise: Diffusion Tensor Imaging Identifies Chronotype-Specificity"; Kenneth Seaton, "Cortisol: The Aging Hormone, the Stupid Hormone," *Journal of the National Medical Association* 87, no. 9 (1995): 667–683.

Habit 3: Start Your Day Right

1. William James, *The Principles of Psychology: Volume I* (1890). York University (Toronto, ON), Classics in the History of Psychology online database, psychclassics.yorku.ca/James/Principles.

2. Vagbhata, *Ashtanga Hridayam, Volume I*, trans. K. R. Srikantha Murthy (Near Golghar: Krishnadas Academy, 2001), 2:1, Scribd.

3. Kabir, *One Hundred Poems of Kabir*, trans. Rabindranath Tagore (Book Jungle, 2007), 32.

4. Christopher Bergland, "25 Studies Confirm: Exercise Prevents Depression," *Psychology Today*, October 23, 2013, psychologytoday.com/us/blog/the-athletes-way/201310/25 -studies-confirm-exercise-prevents-depression.

5. Jalal al-Din Rumi, "Enough Words?" from *The Essential Rumi: New Expanded Edition*, trans. Coleman Barks (New York: HarperOne; Reprint Edition, 2004), 20.

Habit 4: Bestir Your Breath-Body

1. H. Guiney and L. Machado, "Benefits of Regular Aerobic Exercise for Executive Functioning in Healthy Populations," *Psychonomic Bulletin & Review* 20, no.1 (February 2013): 73–86, doi.org/10.3758/s13423-012-0345-4.
2. "Why Do Pranayama?" Kripalu Center for Yoga and Health, accessed October 1, 2018, kripalu.org/resources /why-do-pranayama.
3. *Seinfeld*, episode 86, "The Opposite," directed by Tom Cherones, written by Larry David, Jerry Seinfeld, and Andy Cowan, aired May 19, 1994, on NBC.
4. Eric Grasser, "10 Simple Steps to Wellness . . . ," Dr. Grasser Integrative Medicine & Ayurveda, accessed October 1, 2018, drgrasser.com/blog-1/2014/1/29/protect-promote-project -wellness.

Habit 5: Fuel Yourself with a Plant-Based Diet

1. Katrina Blair, *The Wild Wisdom of Weeds: 13 Essential Plants for Human Survival* (White River Junction, VT: Chelsea Green Publishing, 2014), 49.
2. Philip J. Tuso et al., "Nutritional Update for Physicians: Plant-Based Diets," *Permanente Journal* 17, no. 2: 61–66, doi.org /10.7812/TPP/12-085.
3. Blair, *The Wild Wisdom of Weeds*, 48.
4. "What Is Happening to Agrobiodiversity?" Food and Agriculture Organization of the United Nations, 2004, fao.org /docrep/007/y5609e/y5609e02.htm.
5. "Building on Gender, Agrobiodiversity and Local Knowledge," Food and Agriculture Organization of the United Nations, 2006, fao. org/docrep/009/y5956e/Y5956E00.htm. See also Peter J. Jacques and Jessica Racine Jacques, "Monocropping Cultures into Ruin: The Loss of Food Varieties and Cultural Diversity," *Sustainability* 4, no. 11 (July 21, 2102): 2970–2997, doi.org/10.3390/su4112970.
6. Blair, *The Wild Wisdom of Weeds*, 48.
7. Alex Van Buren, "What's the Deal with . . . Invasivorism?" Yahoo! Lifestyle, April 2, 2014, yahoo.com/lifestyle/whats-the -deal-with-invasivorism-81502314588.html.

Interlude: How to Evolve Your Habits in Relationships
1. Letter from Albert Einstein to Robert Thornton, PhD, December 7, 1944, EA 61-574 in "Einstein's Philosophy of Science," Stanford Encyclopedia of Philosophy website, Stanford Center for the Study of Language and Information, February 11, 2004.
2. Vasant Lad, *Textbook of Ayurveda, Volume 1: Fundamental Principles* (Albuquerque, NM: Ayurvedic Press, 2002), 280.

Habit 6: Self-Massage Your Body
1. Vaidya Bhagwan Dash and Ram Karan Sharma, *Caraka Samhitā, Volume 1* (Delhi: Chawkhamba Sanskrit Series Office, 2015), 88–89.
2. Pat Thomas, "Behind the Label: Nivea Moisturising Lotion," *Ecologist*, June 1, 2005, theecologist.org/2005/jun/01 /behind-label-nivea-moisturising-lotion.

Habit 7: Sit in Silence
1. The Yoga Sutras (sutras 1.47–1.50), translated by Swami Jnaneshvara Bharati, accessed October 1, 2018, swamij.com /yoga-sutras-14051.htm.
2. Yi-Yuan Tang et al., "Short-Term Meditation Increases Blood Flow in Anterior Cingulate Cortex and Insula," *Frontiers in Psychology* 6, (February 26, 2015): 212, doi.org/10.3389 /fpsyg.2015.00212.
3. Talya Dagan, "Meditation Builds Brain Cells, Harvard Study Shows," *Natural News*, February 4, 2015, naturalnews .com/048499_meditation_brain_cells_stress.html.
4. Rebecca Gladding, "This Is Your Brain on Meditation," *Psychology Today*, May 22, 2013, psychologytoday.com /us/blog/use-your-mind-change-your-brain/201305 /is-your-brain-meditation.
5. Jim Loehr and Tony Schwartz, *The Power of Full Engagement* (New York: Simon and Schuster, 2003), 14.
6. James Clear, "How Willpower Works: The Science of Decision Fatigue and How to Avoid Bad Decisions," accessed October 1, 2018, lifehack.org/317884/how-willpower-works-the-science -decision-fatigue-and-how-avoid-bad-decisions.
7. Loehr and Schwartz, *The Power of Full Engagement*, 4.
8. Durant, *The Story of Philosophy*.
9. Loehr and Schwartz, *The Power of Full Engagement*, 181.
10. John Douillard, "15 Benefits of Breathing through Your Nose during Exercise," LifeSpa, May 6, 2014, lifespa.com/15 -benefits-nose-breathing-exercise.

11. "Why Do Pranayama?" Kripalu Center for Yoga and Health, accessed October 1, 2018, kripalu.org/resources/why-do -pranayama.

Habit 10: Live in Ease

1. Craig Hamilton, "Principles of Evolutionary Culture: How You Can Create a Microcosm of 'Heaven on Earth,'" Integral Enlightenment, accessed October 1, 2018, integralenlightenment.com/home/culture.
2. Scott Hauser, "Rediscovering a Lost Spiritual 'Book,'" *Rochester Review* 68, no. 3 (Spring 2006), rochester.edu/pr /Review/V68N3/feature3.html.
3. Hauser, "Rediscovering a Lost Spiritual 'Book.'"
4. Jonathan Fields, *Uncertainty: Turning Fear and Doubt into Fuel for Brilliance* (New York: Penguin, 2012), chapter 4.

There Is No End Game

1. "2.1 Billion People Lack Safe Drinking Water at Home, More than Twice as Many Lack Sanitation," World Health Organization, July 12, 2017, who.int/en/news-room/ detail/12-07-2017-2-1-billion-people-lack-safe-drinking-water- at-home-more-than-twice-as-many-lack-safe-sanitation.

Kitchen Sadhana: Enlightening Your Kitchen

1. N. N. Bhattacharyya, *History of the Tantric Religion* (New Delhi: Manohar, 1999), 174.
2. B. K. S. Iyengar, *Light on the Yoga Sutras of Patanjali* (London: Thorsons, 2002), 22.

Index

foods (*continued*)
  cooking, 213–22
  cravings, 104–5, 168
  and energy, 37–39, 106, 109, 162
  leftovers, 162
  purging, 213–14, 217–18
  staples, 218–20
  superfoods, 107
  see also eating; meals; nutrients;
    plant-based diets
friends. *See* relationships
fruits, 24, 98, 100–101, 105–6, 168,
  171, 176
fulfillment, 77–78, 151
fullness (of stomach), 39–40

gardening (windowsill gardening), 110
genetic erosion, 103–4
Gladding, Rebecca, 150
golden milk, 61
granola, raw buckwheat, 101, 220–21
Grasser, Eric, 88
gratitude, 67, 79, 102
greens, 70, 100–101, 106, 110, 112,
  170–71, 176
ground of being, 198
groups, 9–10, 29, 120, 127

habits, 3–5, 13
  and age, 3–5, 7, 17, 93, 191
  anchor statements, 22–23
  automation of, 28–29
  behavior model, 24–25
  changing, 20, 23–25, 27, 45, 117,
    131–32
  choice architecture, 27–28
  culturing, 13–14
  curiosity, 14
  development of, 13–14
  dinner/supper, 33–49
  easeful living, 193–204
  and environment, 27–28
  evolution of, 13–14, 19–30, 116–18
  goals, 20–21
  and identity, 19–21
  and intention, 15, 23
  kaizen, 23–24

habits (*continued*)
  keystone habits, 29–30
  loop, 25–26
  peer support, 29, 116–20, 126–27
  physiology of, 4–5
  and relationships, 115–32
  and sleep, 58–61
  and stress, 21
  and time, 16, 21
  triggers, 24–25, 35, 44, 117–18
  see also meditation; relationships
Hamilton, Craig, 127, 154–55, 197
hands, as healers, 133–34
hardening exercises, 88–90
headaches, 8, 190
Healthier Eating Guidelines (HEGs),
  163–68
hearing, 186–87
hero's journey, 19–20
holistic medicine. *See* Ayurveda
hormones, 56
human+, 210–11
hunger, 167–68
hydration, 61, 67–70, 79, 161–62,
  167–68, 177

identity, 19–21, 65
immune system, 52–54
  ojas, 57–58
  self-massage, 135
impulse eating, 167
impulsivity, 149, 152
inflammation, 39, 82
information overload, 146–47
insomnia, 60–61
intention, 15
interdependence, 129
invasive weeds. *See* weeds
invasivorism, 111
Iyengar, B. K. S., 214–15

James, William, 23, 72–73
jobs, evening and night, 47
junctures, 18, 190

About the Author

Cate Stillman started Yogahealer.com in 2001 as a bridge for yoga students and teachers to access the wisdom of Ayurveda. She began generating original curriculum when going back and forth between Ayurveda College and a two-year Iyengar Yoga Teacher training. Her two-hour workshop, which she launched in San Francisco in 2000, *Daily Routines of a Yogi*, evolved into this book and the Yoga Health Coaching core curriculum.

Cate has been innovating practical, experiential, evolutionary courses incorporating the wisdom tradition of Ayurveda ever since at Yogahealer. The best way to access Cate and the global Yogahealer community is to listen to her podcast The Yogahealer Real Life Show or to join her email list to receive the many free resources and free trainings at Yogahealer.com.

Cate and her husband are raising their child based in Alta, Wyoming, to ski and mountain bike, and also part-time in Punta Mita, Mexico, to surf and be bicultural. Her cat, Dukha, napped heavily through the creation of this book.

About Sounds True

Sounds True is a multimedia publisher whose mission is to inspire and support personal transformation and spiritual awakening. Founded in 1985 and located in Boulder, Colorado, we work with many of the leading spiritual teachers, thinkers, healers, and visionary artists of our time. We strive with every title to preserve the essential "living wisdom" of the author or artist. It is our goal to create products that not only provide information to a reader or listener, but that also embody the quality of a wisdom transmission.

For those seeking genuine transformation, Sounds True is your trusted partner. At SoundsTrue.com you will find a wealth of free resources to support your journey, including exclusive weekly audio interviews, free downloads, interactive learning tools, and other special savings on all our titles.

To learn more, please visit SoundsTrue.com/freegifts or call us toll-free at 800.333.9185.

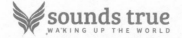

sounds true
WAKING UP THE WORLD